Finding Freedom in Illness

Finding Freedom in Illness

A Guide to Cultivating Deep Well-Being
through Mindfulness and Self-Compassion

Peter Fernando

SHAMBHALA
Boulder
2016

Shambhala Publications, Inc.
4720 Walnut Street
Boulder, Colorado 80301
www.shambhala.com

9 8 7 6 5 4 3 2 1

First Edition
Printed in the United States of America

⊛This edition is printed on acid-free paper that meets the
American National Standards Institute Z39.48 Standard.
♻This book is printed on 30% postconsumer recycled paper.
For more information please visit www.shambhala.com.

Distributed in the United States by Penguin Random House LLC
and in Canada by Random House of Canada Ltd

Designed by James D. Skatges

Library of Congress Cataloging-in-Publication Data

Fernando, Peter, 1976–
Finding freedom in illness: a guide to cultivating deep
well-being through mindfulness and self-compassion/
Peter Fernando.—First edition.
pages cm
ISBN 978-1-61180-263-4 (pbk.: alk. paper)
1. Mind and body therapies. 2. Compassion.
3. Self-care, Health. I. Title.
RC489.M53F47 2016
615.8´51—dc23
2015022877

Contents

Acknowledgments

There are countless people whose presence in my life has contributed to the process of writing this book, both directly and indirectly.

I would like to offer my sincere and deepest thanks to my spiritual teachers and mentors, past and present: Ajahn Sucitto, Sharda Rogell, Ajahn Munindo, Ajahn Amaro, Ajahn Pasanno, Ajahn Viradhammo, Stephen Archer, Ayya Medhanandi, Ajahn Sona, and Ajahn Thiradhammo.

Many of the practices in this book arose directly out of conversations, talks, and advice from Ajahn Sucitto. I would like to acknowledge his significant influence on the themes elaborated in many of the chapters in this book, as well as my exploration of certain Pali words and phrases in a practice context.

Sharda Rogell has been instrumental in guiding me toward a holistic and embodied approach to the Buddhist path. I offer my ongoing gratitude for this, and acknowledge with joy her continued influence on my practice.

Ajahn Munindo's enduring guidance and spiritual friendship has been immeasurably supportive throughout my journey and continues to be so. Many of the perspectives in this book have arisen directly from his teachings and encouragement.

The trainings in somatic awareness presented in this book owe a great deal to the deep wisdom and profoundly loving presence of Garry Cockburn.

Special thanks also to James Baraz, whose compassionate encouragement lit the fire in my heart that led to sitting down and beginning to write; and Stephanie Stewart, whose wise reflections and bright spirit in the face of illness have influenced and inspired the words in this book.

Deep thanks to my spiritual colleagues and friends: Erin Taylor, Hugh Tennent, Jeremy Cole, Lynda Miers-Henneveld, Will Fenton, Kelly Fisher, Melissa Billington, Kara-Leah Grant, Zoe Wild, Marianne Elliott, Kanya Stewart, Billy McGrath, Lena Cromartie, Tracy Williams, Wilhemeena Monroe, Katherine Tate, Nick Potter, Roger Livingstone, Andrew Morrison, Lindsay Alderton, Alys Titchener, and Katie Benge, whose presence has and continues to nourish and deepen my understanding of the path in so many ways.

My heartfelt thanks to everyone who so generously gave their time and energy in assisting me during my years of sickness while in the monastic sangha. In particular I would like to mention Ajahn Ahimsako, Debbie Stamp, Ginger Vathanasombat, Tina Tunyong, Adam Kane, Brian Baumann, Aaron Remmington, Somadevi Ankers, Scott Boultinghouse, Chris Bradley, Stephen Burnell, Sucinno Vermeltfoort, Dave Wakeling, Sister Mon, Stephen Roehrig, Ajahn Pavaro, Dave Gardiner, and Ajahn Jotipalo.

I would like to thank John McArthur for inspiring me with his grace and courage in the face of serious illness, Arna Gaby for her great generosity in welcoming me into her home at exactly the right time, and Dr. John McMenamin for being the most attentive and compassionate doctor imaginable.

Acknowledgments

I offer a heartfelt bow of gratitude to Landa van den Berg and Rutger Keijser for their profoundly generous support, which among many other things enabled me to spend several months in retreat writing this book.

I would like to offer my sincere thanks to Dave O'Neal, my amazing editor, for suggesting that a book may be possible, offering me a koan to sit with, and being so totally supportive and generous throughout the process. I am truly grateful to know you.

Deep thanks to my wonderful family: Jana, Noel, Jan, Julie, and Shelli, for everything you have given me that I can't even fathom. Huge love and gratitude to you.

And lastly, to my beautiful partner, Brighde—without your miraculous love, support, feedback, and deep listening, none of this would even exist.

Finding Freedom in Illness

Introduction

There is a way of relating to illness that takes us directly to the experience of freedom. It is a way of peace, of awakening, and of deep self-kindness. It invites us to become our own best friend and to inquire into the nature of the present moment with freshness, curiosity, and courage. It doesn't involve being anything other than we are right now. This way hinges upon the power of *presence*. Presence, or here-and-now awareness, is the imageless, timeless dimension of ourselves that is always right here behind the conditions of our body and the stories of our mind. When we reconnect with this innate awareness, we remember in our heart that we are always whole, always unconditionally valuable. We awaken to the beauty and strength of self-kindness and compassion. We realize that what we really are, in our heart of hearts, is not an individual who is to blame for our health failing or our body being in pain. What we are is more profound and yet more simple than any image we have of ourselves. This innate sense of presence is the source of our real wisdom and compassion. It doesn't exclude our everyday sense of self, but it also knows that its images and self-definitions are not ultimately true. It can include all of the feelings and sensations of the body and is spacious enough to directly sense their ephemeral, ever-changing nature—loving enough not to tighten around or harden against them through judgment or blame. Whenever we can trust in this simplicity and directness, the experience is one of great relief.

Looking at your human life, your illness, or your challenges from this perspective is inherently liberating, and it doesn't require you to figure out why you are ill or why conditions are the way they are—nor does it require a belief in a future when everything will be the way you want it to be or forcing yourself to be positive so that you won't be sick anymore. The well-being it points to is more simple and innate than all that, and it arises from relaxing wholeheartedly into this very moment right now. It points to an inherent OK-ness in your heart and mind itself that doesn't change in the face of the ebb and flow of health and sickness, pain and pleasure, loss and gain. On a pragmatic level, it is what remains when you let go of all self-judgment, all inner harshness and division, and all dependence on stories and perceptions to define yourself. What is left is what is really true, always.

I have been living with chronic illness for most of my life. My earliest memories of bodily life are of being in a world of wonder, light, and happiness, alongside feelings of great discomfort and the agony of severe eczema that covered my body from the shoulders down. Physical irritation and dis-ease were constant companions, and several times a day I was forced to interrupt my childhood activities with the painstaking ritual of applying thick layers of medicinal creams over my arms, legs, chest, and back, to temporarily allay the endless flaking of skin and excruciating itching. For many years my hands looked almost reptilian, mottled with the scars and discoloration of continuous peeling and cracking. Over time the intensity of the symptoms decreased and the daily experience of my body became more tolerable and free from discomfort. However, in my early twenties, other more invisible and debilitating conditions arose and took my experience of life to new depths of challenge and difficulty. Unrelenting exhaustion, pain, and a severely limited ability to digest food became my daily experience of the physical realm. Generally speaking these conditions matched the symptoms of dysautonomia, gastroparesis, and myalgic encephalomyelitis. Adding to these frustrations was the fact that no single cause could be discerned—all of a sudden I was just really sick. While much healing has taken place, these phenomena still manifest in varying degrees in my daily experience of being alive.

Right now you may be thinking "Wow, that's miserable," but in actual fact, my life has been wonderful so far. When I say "wonderful," I don't mean according to an idea of how life is supposed to look or the "perfect life" that gets sold to us in slick advertisements. Life has certainly been filled with great challenges and loss I would never have asked for, phases of deep darkness and despair, depression, and intense discomfort on the physical level—but with the help of many great teachers and loving friends, the mysteries of being have continued to unfold and reveal an amazing new perspective on what it means to be alive.

In many ways, physical illness has been my greatest, most exacting teacher, and continually asks me to look honestly, compassionately, and clearly into the suffering and confusion I create in the present moment. While I didn't ask for this teacher, nor would I have personally chosen to live with such bodily conditions, they arrived anyway. I could have chosen to see the condition of the body as an enemy rather than a teacher, and I do in many moments. But to live my life from that state would be misery. It has never felt worth it. Instead, I have found that the experience of illness can be a great opportunity to wake up out of the mind's habitual patterns and the limitations and suffering they impose on my awareness and my heart. It is an initiation of sorts. It can take us right into the heart of how we create suffering on top of the here-and-now experience of sickness or disease in the body. As we will see later in the book, suffering and illness are not one and the same.

Some days I find myself sitting in front of my computer holding my head in my hands, with a brain exhausted and swirling, unable to think, my nose dripping nonstop with flulike systems that arrive for no reason, and I remember to just get quiet for a few moments. If I listen, it is like I am being told, "Man, you're caught up in stories. Come back, come back to what's true." In the midst of the shutdown of my faculties and the discomfort of the body, a space opens up—first in my mind's eye, then in the center of my chest—and I reconnect to awareness itself. Relaxing out of the self-images of "Oh, no, I am failing again," and predictions about the future, such as "This day is a write-off," I return to the timeless dimension of being that is always here, behind the apparent reality of the mind's judgments and conclusions. The feeling that this moment is a problem gradually fades and gives way to what always seems like a revelation no matter how many times I return to it: everything is fine. I am fine. These conditions are fine. I can relax.

My journey as a Buddhist monk, which lasted from my early twenties until shortly after my thirtieth birthday, was indispensable to how I gradually learned to use the challenges and discomfort of the body to deepen my longing for freedom. In fact, I don't know how I would have survived without my teachers' help. I spent the first few years in the quiet, simple monastic setting trying to push past the illness of the body and "get enlightened" so that I wouldn't have to deal with it anymore. Through a process of what seemed like endless humiliation, this naive and ultimately egoistic attitude gradually (and often painfully) turned into a more humble approach, as I learned the wisdom of

4

self-compassion, embodied awareness, and a heartfelt acceptance of the present moment.

The compassionate, nonjudging presence of my three main teachers, Ajahn Viradhammo, Ajahn Pasanno, and Ajahn Amaro, all Western monks who trained with the great Thai Forest master Ajahn Chah in the 1970s, mirrored back to me the possibility of relating to myself just as I was, illness and all, in that same way. They showed me how self-compassion and wisdom are intrinsically connected, and they taught me the great value of meeting my experience in as direct, nonjudging, and intimate a way as possible. Through their example as human beings I was shown what a life of integrity, deep kindness, and inner freedom can look like. Over time my willful, individualistic attitude slowly began to break open and I reconnected with the very human need to receive, to reach out, and to be connected to the love and presence of others. Seemingly relentless failure and breakdown on the physical level gave me no choice but to surrender and allow myself to be held in a web of interconnectedness. Later in the book we will explore the importance of this capacity to reach out and allow ourselves to receive love. Like myself, many of you will have been brought up with the idea that we don't need anyone else, that we can do it all on our own. One of the blessings of chronic illness is that it brings it home to the heart that we can't. In fact, no one can. In our habituated cocoon of self-concern we may imagine we can—but really it is just because we don't see how we are already held. Opening into this feeling of being held by others is essential for our well-being as humans, I believe. It allows the most beautiful expressions of the human heart to flow forth—qualities like gratitude, graciousness, and a transparency on the relational level that nourish ourselves and the world around us. When we see these in others, something deep within us recognizes immediately: "Ah, that's what being human is all about. That's what really matters." These qualities can't arise when we are defended, suspicious, and walled off from other people. Nor can they arise if we are walled off from ourselves, our bodies, and the direct experience of our life in the present moment.

This book will offer you practical guidelines grounded in time-honored teachings to awaken your own capacity for freedom and transformation right in the middle of your life and the conditions of your body as they are. Although my main training has been in the teachings of early Buddhism, my interests have been far-reaching, and I draw from many other influences, such as contemporary teachings on somatic awareness and the teachings of wise beings from many other contemplative schools and time periods. You will learn ways of becoming intimate with your own experience of illness or pain in a way that liberates rather than crushes you. In order to achieve this, you will be offered a map to understand how your storytelling mind works, how it creates suffering, anguish, and heart-pain, and how to unfold its patterns in a way that reconnects you to your own capacity for deep self-compassion and freedom of heart. Most important, you will learn how to access the liberating power of here-and-now awareness and to bring it to bear on your experience of sickness, pain, or disability. This awareness, which never leaves us, is both the source of true well-being and the most effective tool in freeing ourselves from habitual patterns of relating to life that obscure the treasures waiting underneath the way things appear to be.

1

You're Not Wrong
for Being Ill

A LOT OF POPULAR thought and teachings these days suggests that if you're ill, it's because you are doing it to yourself—it's kind of *your fault*. When you pick up this belief, painful feelings of guilt and shame quickly follow, along with stories such as "If I were a spiritual person, I wouldn't be ill." This spiral of self-blame serves to increase rather than decrease the pain in your heart and very often the severity of the conditions of your body. While this energy of mind can often come disguised as wisdom or reason, it is actually a kind of self-harm that alienates you from your real potential for well-being. Although the stories it tells sometimes can seem noble or determined, the energy of guilt is itself a form of inner violence. It can very quickly make you more unwell in your body, mind, and heart. Getting clear about this activity of mind is the essential foundation for freeing the heart within the experience of being physically ill. In essence the message is simple: don't beat yourself up for what is happening to your body. It is never worth it.

TWO KINDS OF WELL-BEING

Viewing illness as "un-spiritual" often arises out of the innocent assumption that only one kind of well-being is worth having: physical health. Being spiritual means being physically healthy, and because you are not, you have failed. The idea of living with illness then seems undesirable, a tragedy of some kind, and lamentable. Of course it can feel like all these things on the face of it—but if you're living with illness every day, giving power to these assumptions makes your situation feel unbearable and unworkable. It also sets up a dynamic that will ultimately make both the experience of your illness, and very likely its actual physical symptoms, much worse: resistance to the present moment. Illness then takes us away from presence rather than toward it.

The natural result of only having physical health as a touchstone for well-being is that when it isn't present, when we are in pain, discomfort, or fatigue, we resent our situation and beat ourselves up for it. We resist it. This resistance is what our ego does when all of its attempts at control have failed. So the least it can do, it feels, is fight against what's here. That gives us a feeling of some control but ultimately sows the seeds for more suffering and pain.

This resistance will then influence the way you seek help, through therapies, strategies, or even mental techniques. While there are many therapeutic modes that will be of real benefit on your healing journey, the energy of *seeking* itself can become a source of suffering if it carries the energy of "I am wrong" or "I hate myself for being sick." If your physical condition improves, you will still be divided in your heart and you won't be able to taste the deeper kind of ease and wellness that comes through resting in openness to the continually changing landscape of the present moment. And if you don't get better, everything begins to seem much worse and the feelings of failure and self-criticism take over in crippling ways. Searching for remedies, researching our illness, and seeing health professionals are always more fruitful if instead they come from an undivided state in ourselves. When we relax and unfold beliefs about our own unworthiness or how our illness is evidence that we have failed, our own intuitive faculties are more available to guide us toward what will really be of benefit. Regardless of the outcome, if our heart is open, caring, and informed by our own sense of inherent value, this will serve our aspiration for well-being rather than take us deeper into despair and inner criticism.

This is a spiritual orientation in the deepest sense—it is turning toward that which is always whole, behind the stories of "me and my life," the pasts that could have been and the futures that might not be, right here into the openness and simplicity of being. You could refer to it as the peace that lies within the timeless present. This kind of well-being is the one spoken of by contemplatives throughout history—those who have sought for that which is most intimate, behind the complexity of the ego-mind, and free from identification with the conditions of our life. Perhaps you too have picked up this book because of your own hunger to reconnect with this dimension of being. When we are chronically ill or living in ongoing pain and discomfort, the need to find this inner refuge becomes very compelling.

BEYOND BELIEF

In the course of your experience of living with illness, there may be those who suggest that you are ill because you just don't believe you can be well. Although this kind of advice is often motivated by the desire to help, it can very easily leave you feeling dejected. Not only are you ill, but you are also failing to think the right things. This idea, stemming from the conceit that we are in ultimate control of conditions, is another cause for feelings of inadequacy or self-blame to arise in our heart and mind.

It is very compelling to imagine that if you just thought in a different way you would suddenly get better. In the West we seem to gravitate toward anything that suggests that we as individuals are in total control of conditions. We feel we should be able to be exactly who and how we want to be. This belief underlies much of our discourse, including many contemporary teachings on spirituality and self-help. I am sure many of you have used techniques of positive thinking to try to manifest the conditions you want and fix your illness. I certainly have. However, if we give all of our faith to a need for things to be different, we set ourselves up for the flipside. If conditions remain the same, we feel defeated. When we run out of willful energy, the self-judgments and self-blame of a contracted heart resurface again. You can't have one without the other. They both exist in the realm of the storytelling mind and don't get to the heart of the matter.

The very act of clinging to a belief about how we "should" be or a story about what the illness of the body means "I have done wrong" gives rise to a contracted state of being. This clinging is a very effective way of generating suffering and pain in the present moment. Letting go of this conceit that we have done something wrong (and the assumption that we *should* be in ultimate control of conditions) softens our heart and allows us to come back to a much simpler state of being. Releasing the clinging around these self-judgments is the work of the present moment. Rather than generating more stress and dissatisfaction with our life, it brings about a sense of relaxation and ease around conditions just as they are. From this place we can explore the experience (and perhaps causes) of illness for ourselves.

THE CONTRACTED SELF

The word *contraction* can be used in various ways. I want to clarify what I mean by this and how it relates to the experience of freedom, or its absence, in the midst of sickness, pain, limitation, and exhaustion. On the most basic level, it is that within our mind and body which feels squeezed, closed, or tight. It is the sense of "me" that feels like a failure, broken, unworthy, or useless when we are ill. It's that tight, contracted feeling wedded to images and ideas of ourselves in the mind's eye, which spawns tales of inadequacy, sometimes obvious, sometimes insidious and subconscious. This contracted state also gives rise to the opposite: feelings of superiority, aggrandizement, and invulnerability. Although this side of the mind can and will arise in the process of living with illness, the main focus of this book will be its more obviously painful and limiting expression. In my own experience, and from many conversations with others who experience ongoing illness or disability, it is these stories that pose the greatest challenge to our inner well-being in the midst of pain and limitation.

It is easy to believe that the feelings and thoughts that arise from the contracted state are true. This is the default setting of the human mind, and it comes very naturally to us. To question this assumption takes courage, clarity, and a deep kind of trust. This trust is the feeling sense of your deepest wisdom. It is that which knows you aren't wrong, because what you really are is deeper than any definition, any judgment at all. You could say it's the wisdom of the heart. Or the trust in the awakened mind. Ultimately it is beyond definition, and yet it is the most precious and sacred potential we have.

Throughout this book I use the terms like "storytelling mind," "contracted self," and "ego-mind" interchangeably.

They all refer to the same area of activity in our human hearts and our human being-ness. In essence this activity is the kaleidoscope of mental and emotional fabrication and feeling that arises when we identify with conditions as being "me." When we are sick it often goes like this:

My body is ill→My body shouldn't be this way→*I* shouldn't be this way→It's my fault→I am wrong for being ill.

The thoughts that follow stem from the belief that what you ultimately are is the body and its conditions, and that it essentially defines you. This is a painful state to be in.

The contracted self has two dimensions: the first is the realm of images and ideas, usually concerned with a story about the past or a future or judgments (which are also stories) about ourselves in the present. The second dimension is a *feeling* component, which arises in the present-moment sense of the body itself. This feeling dimension of activity is often experienced on the somatic level as a tightening up, and with it arise the accompanying energies of despair, anger, self-hatred, depression, sadness, despondency, unworthiness, and so on.

So to understand the tendency toward contracted states is to develop both a clarity around the patterns of thought that arise—the stories, beliefs, self-judgments—and a proficiency in bringing awareness right into the here-and-now experience of our body, mind, and heart. The activity of mental turbulence often arises in a finger-snap, so we need to cultivate a presence that is all-encompassing. Sometimes it's in the head, but more often than not, it's a contraction and a feeling in our bodily awareness.

WHAT DO YOU KNOW FOR SURE?

When we enter directly into the awareness that is always here and now, we realize that we don't know. This isn't doubt, which doesn't know but thinks it should—rather, it is acknowledging that we don't know and being at ease with that fact. This kind of not-knowing, in its positive sense, leads to a heart-feeling of relaxation that you can feel in the center of your chest or an unfolding and softness in your belly. It is a beautiful feeling of release from the tyranny of endless wondering and speculation that comes with long-term illness—thoughts such as "Why is this happening to me?" "What did I do to deserve this?" "What have I done wrong?" and "When will this go away?" That kind of seeking to know on the level of thought and ideas is innocent enough, yet it can very quickly generate an undercurrent of stress and dis-ease in your whole body. Relaxing it is a wonderful experience and quite naturally amplifies the sense of presence itself. An openness, a wonder, even.

However, this doesn't mean that you can't or shouldn't take practical steps to get better by taking medicine, seeking advice, or understanding how your lifestyle, choices, or life experiences have contributed to your body's being sick. These are always advisable. Yet you can learn to unhook this kind of everyday knowing from a deeper craving to know *absolutely*. This desire to know can manifest as the question "Why me?" for example, and drive you crazy. But the deeper you look, the more this question becomes unanswerable, and the more you will feel a call to let go of the contracted, unsettled state it generates in the body and mind.

There is a wonderful example of these two levels of knowing in the early teachings of the Buddha, dating from around 600 B.C. I love how they were reflecting deeply on these things even back then. In the discourse to Sivaka, he describes a series of factors that lead to illness and are independent of the volitional activity of mind—or karma, if you choose to look at it like that—forces in nature that are subtle and cause illness as a result of us having these vulnerable human bodies. And after listing these forces, he acknowledged, "Sometimes it's related

13

to karma." *Karma,* it is important to understand here, refers to the results of ways of thinking, being, and acting that come from certain underlying resonances of mind or flavors of heart. It doesn't refer to some force "out there" punishing us, or any sense of being a "bad person." When the Buddha used this word, he actually just meant "cause and effect on the level of mind." The teaching on karma in its most pragmatic sense is optimistic—it opens the possibility for new ways of being, such as those you will learn in this book, and rests upon the freedom to choose how we want to relate to each moment. It isn't about willfully trying to control or manipulate conditions, though. That mind-set generates a causal chain that serves to solidify contracted ways of being rather than dissolve them.

In his lifetime the Buddha encouraged people to take care of their bodies and to look after them in as best a way as they could but never to feel guilty or somehow ultimately to blame for their condition. From the present-moment karmic point of view, guilt is nothing other than self-violence. Reading these texts, you get a sense of the Buddha encouraging his students to realize that "bodies get sick, that's just the way of things." This perspective can open us out of the stories that the mind tells us, which often seem so very personal, unique, and individual, and into a much vaster, universal perspective: this is what happens to bodies sometimes. Indeed, the Buddha's own spiritual path is said to have arisen from his first real encounter with illness, old age, and death. Being a prince of the Sakya clan in northern India, it is said that he was quite sheltered from having to see the raw reality of bodies consumed with illness and disability, bent over with old age, or lying dead. Yet when he reached his late twenties, he was naturally curious and decided to venture out of the confines of this refined and isolated environment. When he wandered out of the palace gates, he was met with this reality in a confronting way—so much so that he described it as a kind of shock to the system. Of course ancient India was nowhere near as sanitized as the streets of a modern city, so one can imagine that all aspects of human life were there in full view. Rather than leading to numbness or despondency, however, this experience of shock turned into a burning desire. It was a wake-up call to find a real refuge amid the fragility of conditions and life on earth itself. As one of my teachers said to me early on, "The Buddha wasn't afraid to lay all the cards on the table." So rather than an idealistic philosophy that says "You shouldn't get ill" and posits some kind of ideal realm where everything *should* be wonderful on the level of conditions, the Buddha's path and teaching arose in relation to the facts of life as they are. These bodies are vulnerable and ultimately out of our own personal control. All of us have to leave them one day. Getting real about this saves us a lot of unnecessary confusion and personal blame for the way things are.

However, this does not mean becoming apathetic or uninterested in what you may be doing to make yourself sick or healthy. On the contrary, you need to be very interested in what is going on in each present moment, in your mind, body, and heart, and in your lifestyle choices. But not from a place of guilt or through attacking yourself with self-judgment. In this way there is no conflict between finding your real home in presence, undefined by conditions of the body and the pragmatic desire to be physically healthy. The former doesn't limit our ability to have a loving and practical relationship to bodily health, while the latter doesn't have to become the measurement of our well-being and value.

DOES THE MIND AFFECT THE BODY?

Having read this far, you may be wondering whether I am suggesting that the activity of your mind has no bearing on your physical health or illness. However, that is not the case. What is not useful is to give energy to feelings of self-blame, guilt, or shame. They will only harm you and serve to cloud your real intuitive wisdom in the present moment. So from the perspective of curiosity and presence, it is beneficial to contemplate how the here-and-now activity of your mind, your emotions, and your attitude affects your whole state of being. This includes your mood, your sense of self, the feelings and sensations in your body, and sometimes the actual physical symptoms of illness or pain themselves. From the perspective of awareness, though, you aren't looking to control experience to get a particular result (the one your mind tells you is most desirable). Nor are you looking to contract around a sense of "It's my fault," or willfully try to get rid of your illness. Rather, you are embarking on a journey right into the present moment, beginning with the feelings and sensations that are here for you, uniquely, right now. It is a process of relaxation, curiosity, and courageous receptivity. As it unfolds, you may encounter habits of mind, such as resistance and unfelt rage or fear, that are contributing to decline of your state of physical health. But regardless of whether or not negative states turn out to be influencing the physical dimension, they are most definitely obstructing the well-being that is most valuable—that of tasting true peace, the simple presence waiting behind all ideas, feelings, and self-judgments.

THE FORCES OF CONSUMER CULTURE

It's also very useful to reflect upon how the culture we live in influences our relationship to physical illness. The values of consumer culture can easily condition our own beliefs about what it means to live within a body that is sick, exhausted, or in pain. Images of the "perfect body" are plastered on enormous billboards, on the covers of magazines, on the back of buses. Illness and death are taboo. So it's not that surprising that we internalize the idea that "this should not be happening." *Should* is the key word here. We can easily become entranced in ideas of how our body "should" be to be "normal."

But what *is* normal—what is real? We don't have to look far—on our street, in our city, to see that human bodies are imperfect. That's their nature. Young bodies age. Healthy bodies eventually get old, get sick, and die. Maybe this isn't "wrong," after all. Maybe these are the cycles of nature itself.

Our culture is also highly performance based. Those who are valued are those who have achieved a lot on the external level. Achievement, production, output—these are seen as what gives us value. But if people are valued for what they have done alone, and not *how* they did it or *who* they are as people in the world, our ideas of value become very limited. So the person who is bedridden or can only just make it out to buy some groceries because they're so exhausted must be failing in some way. Because it doesn't *look* impressive. But in reality, that person (who could be you) may be manifesting beautiful qualities of heart in their encounters and may have a deep peace and self-awareness. When it comes down to it, those are the things that really matter in life.

2

Embodying Mindfulness

IN THE WEST we are trained to live in the world of ideas and thoughts and in our analytical minds. Very little emphasis is placed on cultivating an awareness of our feelings or developing an intelligence that spans the emotional as well as the conceptual. Many of us can progress into adulthood with very developed intellectual faculties but a sorely undeveloped capacity to connect with the feeling quality of our embodied life in the present moment.

To fully taste the benefits of awareness and the power of relating to our illness, pain, or fatigue from the perspective of presence, we need to become open to the possibility that awareness is far more than just a faculty of the cognitive mind—it is in fact all-encompassing and can be present for our entire body, our deepest feelings, and our most intimate sense of self. Awareness, that presence that we are, in not just located in the head somewhere between our eyes. On the most fundamental level it is also that which *feels*—it is the sensitivity that receives the impressions of sound, taste, smell, sight, and perhaps most important in working with physical illness, touch. The realm of the tactile, the directly sensed feeling of the body here and now, becomes a doorway for a more subtle capacity of awareness: feeling the presence of the body from the inside out.

This capacity to develop an embodied feeling-awareness becomes essential when we are in a state of ill health, discomfort, or pain. Although it seems counterintuitive—perhaps like the last thing you would want to do—it is in fact the only place you can transform, heal, and unfold your relationship to the gritty, unpleasant sensations themselves. From the thinking mind, or even a clear space of awareness in our heads, we still remain dissociated, and the mind's present-moment expression in the body, as resistance, tightness, clenching, or a habitual defended-ness, remains hidden. When these deeper expressions of mind are hidden, pain, discomfort, and fatigue will feel much more intense. They become perceived as "unbearable," and an attitude of defiance and ill will can take over our mind and heart.

Cultivating an embodied awareness doesn't mean becoming masochistic, however—it's not a matter of just "facing your pain." That attitude is also disconnected from a genuine heart of self-kindness and compassion and will wear you out very quickly. The art is to gradually become aware of the felt sense of your relationship to the condition of your body in this very moment. The point isn't to focus on or amplify the unpleasant sensations but to connect to the here-and-now effects of your intentions and attitude in a way that empowers you and gives you the choice of whether to sustain them or to relax, soften, and feel for a new possibility entirely.

CURIOSITY AND OPENNESS

Curiosity is essential when it comes to learning an embodied approach to mindfulness. In my early years of meditation practice,

I recall often finding myself at a kind of precipice, in between being completely lost in the storytelling mind and actually contacting the felt sense of the body with awareness. It was as if I had come across a very old wall in the heart and mind that prohibited access to a full feeling of the body. Getting curious about this, I began to gently keep my attention on the sensations and reactions that arose whenever I inclined my attention toward feeling my belly or my chest. This curiosity was and is a kind of inner listening. I found myself listening to the the reactions that deflected attention and spun the mind into streams of thought—giving them all the time in the world and becoming very interested in gently returning to the position of mindful awareness, over and over again.

Becoming curious in this way led to a gradual reeducation of the feeling intelligence of awareness itself. Being present for the process of resistance occurring underneath the surface of the storytelling mind, I was able to see a chain of cause and effect that had been hidden. Directly feeling the causes of the body-mind contraction in a space of nonjudgmental awareness was a kind of revelation. I realized how much worse I had been making myself feel every time my heart closed up and I gave strength to the stories and energy of anger and hate. The possibility of relaxing these habits became enticing.

"What would it be like to just allow myself to feel this way?" I asked myself. "You mean, just this way? Exactly as I am?" the mind would ask back. "Yeah, just exactly how you are—however that is." What arose then were feelings of trepidation, fear, and a subtle protective energy of shame. This feeling of shame was very interesting to me, as it came as a total surprise. "What's this about?" I wondered, and just allowed awareness to listen for the stories.

"You can't just feel how you are!" I heard myself say, from deep down. "Oh, why not?" I asked back from the position of curious awareness. "Well . . . that's dangerous," the heart replied.

"It's, you know . . . it's bad!" Discovering this assumption in my heart was a huge "aha" moment. I had finally contacted something deep within myself that had been very good at hiding from awareness. It was a primal shame around feeling *itself*—a mistrust of being in the body. As I gently unpacked the assumption, it began to reveal more biases that it had inherited from what seemed like a long time ago: "The body is shameful. The body is messy. The body is stupid. You need to get it together, man. Take control. . . ." Being able to hold these painful and tragic assumptions in awareness was a gradual process that involved a relaxing of the desire to push past them (more willfulness) as well as sustaining the energy of a kind and loving curiosity about the effects of this assumption in the present moment. Meeting and unfolding this shame response was for me a key part of learning to access a direct embodied awareness and being able to taste the resulting experience of wholeness.

What you find when you begin this inquiry will be unique to yourself and your situation. My aim in describing the process above is just to give you a feel for how the inquiry can unfold; it is in no way meant to suggest or preempt what you will meet. Indeed, you will need to have as open and curious an attitude as possible—being clear that you don't know and that you are just interested in exactly what is here right now in the direct experience (underneath your stories and ideas) of your body and mind. From this nonjudgmental curiosity, aligned with a heart of self-kindness, you will begin to sense yourself in a whole new way. Embodying awareness always feels good, even if what we meet in the process is sensitive, turbulent, or emotionally difficult.

CULTIVATING BODILY AWARENESS

In the teachings of early Buddhism, the word *mindfulness* (*sati* in the Pali language) is often hyphenated with the word *sampa-*

janna, meaning an all-around, full awareness. The ability to witness, to see, and to direct our attention is very useful, as we will explore throughout this book—but if it is to bring about real transformation it needs to be based in the here-and-now experience of the body. We can train ourselves to feel our human heart and mind as a living, ever-changing energy, right here in the body itself.

There are many ways of strengthening and cultivating your inherent capacity to sense this embodied awareness. It is interesting to note that in the meditation teachings of the Buddha, awareness of the body is considered the First Foundation of Mindfulness. This highlights its significance in the journey to inner well-being, freedom, and insight. For many of you, the journey I spoke of above may sound inviting, but you may also be wondering where to begin. Indeed, I have often heard people respond to the notion of feeling whole in the body with a mixture of bemusement and interest, followed by a statement such as "I can't even feel my body."

In many ways, living with a chronic illness is already an enormous advantage. You are forced, despite your wishes, to attend to the living reality of bodily life on a daily basis. The restrictions, malfunctions, and unpleasantness of the body keep calling you back to the present moment, even though you would, naturally, wish it was otherwise. Yet if you are reading this, you most probably have been faced with the reality that avoiding it altogether is not an option. Perhaps there is a kind of grace in illness in that it yanks us from our fantasy world of the past and future and right back into the present moment. The way you meet this experience of the present moment is what will determine its outcome. Rather than dragging you kicking and screaming, the call to embodiment can become a conscious journey.

The most widely used method of bringing about the direct sense of embodied awareness, especially in the Buddhist tradition, is to place attention on the natural experience of breathing. For many of you, the way your physical illness manifests may affect your ability to engage in a traditional version of the process, so I will suggest a gentler way that has worked for me.

GUIDED MEDITATION:
THE NATURAL RHYTHM OF BREATH

You may want to pause after each instruction that follows and close your eyes to get a sense of feeling-awareness itself. It is also all right to leave your eyes open; if you choose to do so, try to soften your gaze so that you are not focused too intently on the details of what you see.

In the posture you find yourself in right now, become aware of the fact that you are breathing. Just feel the breath wherever it feels pleasant, accessible, and free from discomfort or pain. There's no need to strain to focus on the breath as an object that you need to grab on to. Instead, let the gentle rhythm of breath become conscious as a direct experience in the field of bodily presence itself. There is only one important thing to keep in mind: don't think it; *feel* it.

Notice your capacity to consciously touch it, feel it, sense it, with a receptive, open awareness. Allow yourself to rest in this receptive quality. Become friendly with the sensations in awareness. How fully can you feel them? Allow your awareness to be held by the gentle rhythm of expansion and contraction undulating through your body. Rest in this natural rhythm. Feel the primal nature of it. You don't have to control it—it is an aspect of nature. It is holding you. Always.

Begin to rest in the whole-body feeling of this rhythm. Feel how your core sense of presence comes alive as you do this. If the mind begins wandering into stories, doubts around "Am I doing it right?" just come back. You *are* doing it right. You are safe here. Just be here in the body. Relax any striving to make any-thing happen or to "go somewhere." Just be here with the breath and rest in presence. Allow the energy that comes from this rest-ing to suffuse the present moment. Drink it in. Savor it. Bathe in it. Relax into it. Let yourself come home into the heart of the moment itself.

You may want to put the book down now and just rest with your breath for however long it feels beneficial.

be of the body

This kind of practice strengthens and galvanizes your ability to be present for the body, and for the effects that a conscious rela-tionship to it bring about. You may have noticed a softening, relaxing, and perhaps uplifting effect on your mind and heart that came from a friendly, open attention to the natural rhythm of your body breathing. This is a key piece of information on your journey to embodied awareness: the way your attention relates to the present-moment experience of the body has a huge effect on your state of inner well-being.

It is important to state here, once again, that we are not try-ing to will a preconceived outcome, physical or mental, into ex-istence. There is no failing or succeeding. Instead, you can enter into the process with a heart-quality of innocence and curiosity. Allow yourself to be that simple. As with all of the practices in this book, your primary orientation is a trust in your inherent wholeness—that your most intimate presence, that which you truly are, is already perfect here and now. Attuning to this trust bears wonderful fruit.

Another practice you can try is what is known as a body scan ✓ meditation. You can do this sitting in a chair or even on the floor. Lying on your back or to one side can be very useful, especially if the condition of your body makes it hard to stay upright. I have used lying down with awareness as a practice for more than a decade, and it can have very fruitful results. One advantage that lying down has is that it relieves the pressure that can build up in the system if your energy is waning and your willpower is required just to stay upright. It can create the feeling of coming home to yourself, particularly if your intention is clearly to connect to presence and a curious, spacious awareness. If you find that sleepiness is a problem, then leaning against a wall or sitting upright in bed may be more useful for you.

At times when your body is not in too much discomfort, lying on your back can be useful in creating a feeling of expansion and spaciousness around the felt sense of the body. However, if the overall experience of your bodily sensations is painful, tight, stuck, or just "yuck," lying to one side can help bring about an experience that feels safe, protected, and almost embryonic. This can help generate a field of kind and caring attention to hold our present-moment experience within. Even a few moments in this posture can feel restorative when we enter it with a clear intention to be aware and awake with a friendliness and warmth toward the experience of the body.

GUIDED MEDITATION: BODY SCAN

For this meditation it can be useful to have your eyes closed, so you may want to ask a friend to read the instructions to you. You can also record yourself reading it and play it back for yourself to listen to when the time feels right.

Coming back to the experience of awareness in the present, settle into a posture that feels comfortable for your body. Begin by wiggling your fingers and toes to reconnect attention with the felt sensations in the present moment. Take a moment to feel the overall quality of feeling that is present for you now. Is it heavy? Is there tightness? Does the body feel light and wispy like a feather? Are there sharp, unpleasant feelings or areas of buzzing restless energy? Whatever you encounter, relax any impulse to judge it, contract around it, or compare it to an ideal of how it should be for a "proper" meditation. Instead, breathe out, soften your attention, and relax with this moment. This moment is not wrong—it is the perfect moment to be here, just as you are.

Now place your attention at the soles of your feet and move it up to your ankles and back down again to your heels. Feel what is there for you. Can you notice the difference between the mental image of "my feet" in your head and the actual sensations that are present in that area of your body right now? You don't need to label them; you just need to connect to them as a direct experience. Is there a tingling? Is there warmth or coolness? You can even move your feet around gently to animate the sensations and make them more tangible in awareness. Again, relax and soften any judgment—you don't need any result here. If sensations are interesting, strong, or vibrant, that is good. If they feel numb, elusive, and vague, that is also good. What matters is your intention to open to feeling-awareness in the present moment. Stay curious. Bring a sense of wonder to your presence. How does it feel to *feel*?

If you encounter strong sensations of pain as you do the scan, remember that you don't have to focus on them, wonder about why they are there, or try to get rid of them. For now, just note their presence and soften the impulse to react or judge. Relax into the awareness of the present moment and allow stories and interpretations to take a back seat.

Move your attention gently and spaciously up through the legs, again coming out of the mind's images and into direct contact with the sensations themselves. Allow your attention to sweep up, down, around your calves, knees, thighs, and pelvic area. Keep it very simple. Feel what is here and stay connected to awareness itself. Feel your awareness sweeping through the cells of the body with kindness and care. Notice if any desires to make healing happen arise in your heart. For now, just relax those too. Allow presence to be as simple and open as possible. How clearly can you feel sensations as sensations?

If your body becomes restless, allow yourself to wiggle a little or even rock back and forth gently. Find a balance between the overall intention to be still and the needs of the body's energy system.

Now sweep your spacious, caring attention over your belly, around to the lower back, the kidneys, then back around again. Feel what is alive here. The rhythm of breath may become conscious again—if so, just let it flow naturally, and enjoy the sensations that arise. If it feels right, you can even bring a smile to your awareness. Sometimes imagining an inner smile helps to soften attention out of habits of resistance and contraction and bring it more in tune with the natural quality of openness and love.

Continue to explore the feelings of the upper body with your awareness. Move up and around the chest, the shoulders, the shoulder blades, and then bring your attention down each arm, one at a time. You may like to play with certain ways of sweeping awareness—such as spiraling or moving up and down in long strokes. The important thing is to stay connected to the sensations of the body themselves and not to get too caught up in trying to make anything happen. The mind loves to make things happen, but resting that impulse allows a deeper dimension of embodied stillness and presence to reveal itself. Through relaxing the need to control, we often experience a new kind of ease and well-being, which permeates and suffuses our aware presence underneath the particular details of sensation.

Now bring your spacious, curious awareness up the neck and around the back of the head, sweeping up, down, and around, feeling what is here for you. Notice the sensations themselves without judgment. Moving around to the face, feel if you can sense how you are holding your expression in this moment. How are your lips? What do your eyelids feel like? Relax the need to hold yourself together and just allow awareness to suffuse the muscles of your face, touching every cell with gentle, warm attention.

Notice the images of "me" that arise in your mind's eye, the image of the person you feel yourself to be, and keep being curious about the experience of direct feeling-awareness underneath them. Sometimes a lot of energy can arise when we bring this kind of attention to our face, as this can be a significant place of holding. When you relax the holding, you may notice other parts of your body becoming energized. This is normal, so don't be surprised if it happens. And even if nothing at all happens, just inclining your attention and intention toward this kind of intimacy with the present moment is the doorway to a new kind of well-being.

AWARENESS BECOMES PRESENCE

As we have seen, it is not enough to have only a cognitive understanding of awareness in the present moment, as the real life of our mental habits is occurring more directly and viscerally in the body itself. Our body is integral to what we feel ourselves to be, so if our attention remains somewhere above the shoulders, we end up missing out on the possibility of profound transformation, not just in how we think but in who and what we feel ourselves to be. When change happens on that level, it affects all the more peripheral levels of our being, such as the quality of thoughts, our everyday sense of self, and how we perceive those around us. We get to the heart of the matter and a new sense of well-being flows forth from that.

In exploring the exercises above, you may have noticed a gathering together of focused attention felt as a heightening of awareness in your body itself. Sometimes it is localized, such as in the center of the chest or the spine; however, when I am experiencing discomfort or pain I have found it useful to also maintain an intention to make it all-encompassing, so that my whole body feels held within a field of kind attention. This home-coming of awareness into a whole body and mind alertness is what allows us to shift from merely thinking about awareness, or "watching" our thoughts, to embodying presence itself. In the old Buddhist texts, consciously exercising the mind in this way is said to bring about an experience called *samadhi*. This Pali word isn't something abstract or remote but rather refers to the intimate experience of being grounded in the here and now and allowing our whole body and mind to rest in a peaceful aliveness away from the incessant stream of inner chatter generated by the thinking mind.

Samadhi is a way of connecting to the energy of awareness itself, so that it becomes a living, vital experience of presence. It has an energetic, felt quality to it, which generates a kind of strength and steadfastness in the center of our being. You could call this the heart center, or our core presence, but in reality it is indefinable and has to be experienced for oneself. It is what happens when our attention isn't being diluted through the currents and obsessions of the thinking mind, with its pasts, futures, concerns, and worries, and instead has come alive in the field of embodied awareness. As we have seen, this awareness isn't something we have to get—it is always here and now. Practices that give rise to the quality of *samadhi* are just ways of animating that awareness so that it becomes the focus of our experience.

When awareness becomes the primary focus of our attention—rather than images, ideas, and our inner chatter—the quality of *samadhi* gathers naturally in the heart. Embodied awareness then becomes a palpable, living experience that refreshes us and returns us home to the heart of the moment. The experience of *samadhi* doesn't depend on the body being healthy, pain-free, or full of energy. While it does suffuse the felt sense of our body, it actually takes place on a level deeper and more intimate than the conditions we are experiencing. We begin to feel ourselves to *be* that and rest in this dimension of mind and heart that is independent of the brokenness, exhaustion, or discomfort our body is experiencing. This is the beauty of it. From this place our presence can then radiate out, meet, and embrace what is here, as we will see in the next chapter.

PRESENCE CAN MEET ALL OF LIFE

The paradox of cultivating the quality of *samadhi* is that it can create a duality in our lives, where we end up trying to get to a state that we once were in and miss out on what is here in the present moment. As a remedy for feeling overwhelmed with mental noise, self-critical mind states, or physical discomfort, it is useful and beneficial, but it becomes very limited if it is our only strategy in the long term, particularly when our body is unwell. If we live in a sense of opposition to our life as it is, we end up valuing the "spiritual bit" and subconsciously devaluing the rest of experience. From the perspective of awareness, however, it is *all* the spiritual bit. It can all be embraced in the field of our wholehearted and curious presence. Even the most beautiful and uplifting meditative states are just that: states. They come and they go. If our ego-mind co-opts these states, then we very quickly find ourselves at odds with the gritty mess of embodied life.

So rather than grasping on to meditative states, we can use the experience of *samadhi* to strengthen our trust in awareness itself and to resonate with all of experience. In the context of a life lived with chronic illness, this is the real blessing that sincere meditation practice can bestow upon our lives. More division and resistance don't help in the long run—even if what we are trying to get to is a memory or an ideal of a spiritual state. And ironically, if we do try to grasp on to special states, one of the first universal truths we learn, sometimes frustratingly, is that the grasping itself is what will push them out of our reach. So we might as well relax into how we are, in this very body and mind, right now.

The challenge, then, is to be able to both enjoy and then let go of the effects of meditative states—the particular by-products of heightening, pleasure, or even feelings of bliss—and use meditation as a means of strengthening our core presence. We do this from a place of non-clinging—an availability for the whole spectrum of the feelings, tones, and textures that human life involves. We can remain curious, open, and in a state of inquiry around what is here, in *this* moment. And this moment. And this one. This is a twenty-four/seven process, and it is where the real transformation and self-knowledge occurs. Taking the strength of awareness that comes from *samadhi* right into the chaotic and unpredictable experience of illness, exhaustion, and feelings of failure or despair shines a light on what exactly we are doing in the present moment to make everything seem "wrong." In our embodied awareness we also begin to feel the quality of contraction that accompanies negative states; we begin to notice what happens when our presence tightens, hardens, and clenches around a sense of "me" in relation to the raw experience of life. Developing *samadhi* gradually increases this capacity of attention and allows us to get very real with our mind and heart in the present. It allows us to come out of a fragmented state of being and right back home to the intimacy of being ourselves in this very moment. The relief that comes from this is far greater than any feeling or state—it is the revelation that we are already home, always. The mind loses its power to kidnap us and take us far away into dark, cramped places where we would rather not be.

So knowing how to find the balance in meditation for oneself is where it's at. We can use the experience of meditative presence to refresh, refuel, and revitalize the heart and mind, while also developing the courage to be here for our life in its visceral, raw suchness. These two work together. The deepest shifts occur when we can meet the patterns of heart and mind as present-moment phenomena that have a quality of life energy to them. That quality of life energy isn't always pleasant, which is the challenge. It is often the very stuff that we have tried not to feel—perhaps for a lifetime. This is what the strength of *samadhi* allows us to gradually meet, with sensitivity, wisdom, and great kindness for ourselves. It is all of that stuff—the residual dark feelings—that has been locked away from our awareness and that has a lot of secret power over the mind. Beginning to open up to that dimension of ourselves is very powerful.

Right now you may be wondering to yourself, "Well, it sounds powerful, but how do I do that?" That is a very good question, and it's one we will look at in the next few chapters. It is important for you to bear in mind that there is no fixed or absolute method for navigating this terrain in yourself—you just have to become interested in it and trust in your own intuition that it is possible to transform affliction into ease. Self-kindness and a commitment to nonjudgment are the foundation for this exploration. Embodied awareness and the power of presence open up a space of strength and steadfastness in ourselves that allows us to begin to hold more of the "stuff" of life in the present moment without being shaken off balance and without becoming caught in compulsive reactivity. We can begin to ask ourselves, "What's going on anyway, right now?" We can slow down enough to begin to feel it.

What drives your patterns of mind? What forces condition your self-images and the habitual ways you perceive yourself?

What energies of heart propel you into fixed ideas of "the future"? How do they affect you? These are the kinds of questions that your own clear and compassionate awareness can begin to ask in the space of presence itself. Slowing down enough to ask these questions in a heartfelt way is already a quiet revolution in your being.

3

From Self-Blame
to Self-Kindness

WHEN FACED WITH illness and physical limitation it is easy
to begin searching for something or someone to blame. While
the desire to understand cause and effect is natural and important, the desire to blame is an unnecessary step in this process.
And yet for many of us it is an often unseen force in the heart
and mind with a lot of unconscious energy behind it. When our
attention becomes caught in this pattern, the first object of
blame it will believe it has found is "me." Rather than attending with objectivity to certain possible causes, the mind then
contracts around guilt and starts to attack our very sense of
self. This mental pattern begins to harm us rather than fulfill-
ing its desire to understand why we are ill. The heart closes and
we begin to foster a state of being that can make our condition
much worse. Thankfully, however, another way of being is
possible. We can begin to open, find a real sense of kindness
toward the whole of our lives, and free ourselves from the tyr-

anny of endless criticism and inner fault finding. When we do this, everything begins to change.

AWARENESS

All of the practices and perspectives offered in this book hinge upon your ability to connect to the immediacy of awareness itself in the present moment. This faculty of attention, of being, may be unfamiliar to you, so it will be useful to explore it in more depth before we begin applying it in certain ways. Later in the book you will learn to go deeper into the quality itself, but for now I will outline the basic principle so that you can explore it in your own present-moment experience. It may be useful for you to pause at certain points, close your eyes, and get a taste of the experience that the words are pointing to.

Awareness is that quality of yourself, right now, that can *know* all of your thoughts, all of your stories, and all the feelings and sensations in the body, as objects. It never goes away and is always right here, and yet it is the first thing we usually overlook. This habit of looking past awareness is just the human condition and nothing to feel bad about. However, you can train yourself to recognize that awareness is here and now and begin to see everything that arises and takes shape, even those stories and self-images that seem very personal and real, in a much vaster context—that of the edgeless space of your own awareness itself. Training yourself in this new way of being can take many forms, as you will see, but the most important factor is your own genuine curiosity, interest, and willingness to see your mind for what it is rather than what it wants you to believe you are and what your illness means.

For example, sometimes I wake up feeling a lot of physical discomfort and fatigue for no reason. Even though I have slept well, and for a good length of time, upon waking the body feels like it has just run a marathon (or been "hit by a truck" as I sometimes more graphically express it). Although this is part of my condition and very familiar, it is often the case that the mind will begin to create stories of failure within minutes of getting out of bed. These stories of failure then give rise to a tight, contracted feeling in the body and a sense of fear and guilt that I can feel in my belly.

I then have two choices. The first is to believe that these stories of "It's my fault" are real, are true, and then live from them. This invariably makes the experience feel much worse. The second is to pause, relax, and notice that this entire state arises in a field of present-moment awareness that is actually quite peaceful and OK. The guilt, the story of "I must have done something wrong to be feeling this bad," the searching into the past to look for evidence of something I have done "wrong," are all objects rippling, changing, and being regenerated in the field of presence itself. That presence isn't defined by those objects of consciousness, nor is it a judgment about them being there in my mind and body. It just is. It is the light, the space, right here at the heart of all experience, underneath the apparent reality of the ego's projections, comparisons, and judgments.

Choosing this second option is a kind of *waking up*. It is recognizing what is real, true, and always the case in this moment. It takes effort and courage, certainly, but it isn't about being willful or straining either. Nor is it trying to force positive thoughts into existence, get on with it, or "stop being so stupid." It is the act of pausing and remembering what is really going on here: my mind is creating a story about what it means to be exhausted and uncomfortable. The story is a construction. I made it up. I don't have to believe it.

The result of relaxing into this sense of presence is a natural loosening up of the power that the associated emotions of guilt and worry have on my mind and heart, and also a clearing up of the confusion that results from identifying with a story of "wrongness" around my sense of self. Through being attentive enough not to collapse into believing the story—*and* relaxed enough to not have to try to get rid of it, the space of awareness reveals itself to be the true meaning of this moment. When I rest there, it blossoms as a deep sense that everything is OK—this fatigue, this discomfort is just the way it is. I don't have to let it define me, and I don't have to dwell in the sense of "my fault." This is the great healing power of awareness itself.

ACCEPTANCE AND RELAXATION

The feeling quality of this present-moment awareness is a heart of acceptance. When you see that this moment is just *this way*—that all of your stories and interpretations are not the actual reality of what is going on—there is a natural relaxation of resistance that occurs. You begin to sense that resistance is itself a state of distress and has the potential to send your mind into turmoil very quickly. Whenever you can taste the openness and spaciousness that unfurls when resistance is released, the experience of being alive becomes much lighter.

Resistance has many levels. The most obvious way it manifests is often in our whole perspective on illness itself, and what it means about the present moment, our lives, and our value. The meaning we give to our entire situation can often become tinged with an underlying sense of "This shouldn't be happening to me." This kind of resistance then filters into more subtle levels of our response to the present moment. Our relationship to our body becomes akin to that of an enemy, an aberration that has let us down. It becomes harder to be with the body as it actually is in this moment. Unpleasant feelings become interpreted as attacks on ourselves, and we react with more negativity in response. This creates a cycle of emotional pain and contraction that amplifies the pain of pain itself. The more we react with ill will and view the present-moment experience of the body through the filter of enemy images, the more it seems to be hurting us deliberately or conspiring against our well-being. Perceiving in this way makes us agitated, confused, and unhappy, and in the end only serves to inhibit the possibility for real healing.

For the first few years after my body had become ill in my twenties, I defaulted into a position of anger and defiance against its condition. I recall saying to myself in private moments, almost unconsciously, "I hate this body." And I felt it. My thoughts would revolve around a kind of bitter resentment for the body having "let me down," and the feelings and thoughts that predominated were along the lines of "How could 'you' [insert expletives directed toward the body] do this to 'me'?" It is painful to remember such harshness, but I am sure you have had similar experiences in your own journey.

In spite of all the apparent strength that I thought would come through this kind of hard-hearted willpower, the condition of the body got worse and worse. It took a few years of continuous defeat, which included my digestive system almost completely failing, to realize that this perhaps wasn't the wisest way to relate to my body—and my life in general. Around this time I remember being alone one morning in a cabin in the frozen Canadian winter, feeling both hopeless and deeply resentful toward the condition of my body. My teacher and mentor, Ajahn Viradhammo, who had come to visit for a few days, generously popped in to see how I was doing. In his compassionate presence, I began to open up about how I really felt, and found myself speaking from assumptions of how "I should feel" and "My body should be" in a candid, unguarded way. He then challenged me, gently and with kindness, on the belief that I should be able to "get over it" through meditation and willpower rather than through actually taking care of myself with compassion.

"What do you think the results of hating the body will be?" he asked. I was taken aback. My self-image was definitely not one of someone who hated his body. However, over the next few days, as his words kept coming back to my heart, it dawned on me, "I am actually really angry. I've made this whole situation into an enemy for my ego to conquer. And it's only getting worse. Maybe I've completely missed the point." It turned out I had.

Through opposing, resisting, and asserting the ego's "shoulds" on my situation, I had become dissociated from the actual experience of the body in the present moment. Instead of meeting the body from the position of awareness, interest, and an appreciation of the mystery of each moment, I was living in rigid ideas and judgments of "my body" and only seeing them. Feelings of pain and discomfort that arose on the feeling level were filtered through an interpretation of "I hate this," while rare moments of relief were judged as "This is right. I want more of this." From this dissociated stance, I had begun to foster a relationship of anger toward the body itself. This lack of embodied awareness, as we will see later, drains what life energy there is left in our system and makes the experience of illness much worse on all levels—mental and physical.

As I softened this resistance, I began to heal the painful gap I had created between my mind and my body. The doorway was in awareness and acceptance—seeing that the judgments and overlaid images of "my sick body" were being fabricated in each present moment, and I could choose to see them as such. Resting in an attitude of acceptance gave awareness a power to question the structures of mind I had normally taken to be real. Opening up my inner experience in this way was a great blessing—I began to be able to see and feel anger and hate *directly* as anger and hate, but stay in awareness and not buy into the story they were spinning. And underneath that, the discomfort and dysfunction of the body could also be received as just that. Not "wrong," or "my fault," but just feeling and sensation themselves. This gradually led to a new kind of well-being that came through a renewed curiosity and a feeling of ease and peace with the body just as it is. I could feel the body relaxing gradually, and while many of the conditions persisted and still do to this day, what unfolded was the peace of being able to feel whole and alive in being itself, regardless of the body's energy levels or physical wellness. This energy of being, of presence, is subtle at first, but gradually begins to permeate the experience of embodiment itself.

It is important to say here that the absence of resistance and the feeling state of acceptance do not imply resignation. It is not a giving up of your ability to make wise choices, to care for the body, and to want to be well. You need those capacities, as your very life energy depends upon them. However, it is a question of what place in your heart you make those choices from. While resistance and the feeling of bitterness, aversion, and their shadow side of victimhood narrow your field of attention and keep you stuck on a hamster wheel of seeking, avoiding, blaming, looking to the past for answers, and praying for a future that looks a certain way, empowered acceptance, grounded in present-moment awareness, frees up your thinking and allows you to be very creative. When your mind is not clouded and obstructed by destructive thoughts and emotions, its real power to choose shines forth. Resting in and trusting the inherent OK-ness of here-and-now awareness also allows you to access deeper levels of intuition and wisdom related to your illness, your life, and relationships as a whole, as we will see later. The benefits are vast.

Resignation, on the other hand, is a collapse into depressive states, such as "Why bother?" or "There's nothing I can do anyway," which have a feeling quality of suffering and darkness to them. It is important not to mistake these for acceptance and awareness. The states that arise from resignation are actually more of the same storytelling mind—the belief in a "me" at the center of the universe—but rather than being all-powerful, this "me" is impotent, hopeless, and weak. Resignation is easy to default into when we have been sick for a long time, so it is important to remember that acceptance does not preclude creative action. Rather than inhibiting well-being, connecting to present-moment awareness and resting in the feeling of acceptance opens the doorway for us to experience the real treasures of contentment, love, gratitude, and profound homecoming that can be found in the heart of the moment itself, even in the midst of physical illness, fatigue, or pain.

BECOMING CONSCIOUS OF YOUR STORIES

When we become interested in the possibility of finding our home in an attitude of acceptance and openness, we simultaneously meet all the stories our minds tell us about the present, the past, and the future. When we are sick, have a disability, or are in chronic pain, these stories may often have the characteristics of self-judgment, shame, comparisons to others, or images of how we "should be." No matter how deeply personal and absolutely true they may seem, these are all stories the mind is creating in the present moment. They are fabrications of mind that condition the feeling of "me" as wrong, unworthy, a failure, or not good enough.

Very often these stories lurk somewhere under the surface, souring our mood, creating a heaviness, tightness, or sense of being inadequate in some way. Can you sense the presence of any of these in your mind right now?

 You may want to pause, put down the book, and just become aware of the content of your mind and the feelings in your body for a moment.

What stories about yourself did you find? Sometimes these may not be obvious, so you have to listen carefully with a spa-

Dana?
mind's view/st?
body
Body Head (full
awareness
of body)

cious awareness. Try listening to your mind as if it were your best friend sharing something secret about him- or herself with you. Lean into the person telling you things in your mind's inner ear, the person we normally identify with as "me," with a gentle, compassionate, and curious attention. You may want to silently ask your mind, "What are you saying?" See if you can become aware of the whole *flavor* of the mind state. Your awareness can do this, like we do with food—but on the more subtle level of the mind and the feelings and emotions it creates in the body.

What thoughts about the past obsess your mind in the present moment? What do they appear to tell you about a "me" that you really are? How does this "me" feel? Good or bad? Successful or useless? At the moment you're just becoming interested in this whole realm of storytelling—the creations of our mind that we so often take for granted and live out of, forgetting the deeper dimension of simple presence underneath. We forget that what we really are isn't any of the self-images our mind is spawning. It is much more direct and simple than all of that.

If you become aware of a particularly harsh story about yourself, it is important not to judge it, try to get rid of it, or blame yourself for "thinking these stupid thoughts." Soften and relax that impulse. Instead, open your field of awareness and listen deeply. Listen to everything your inner voice is saying and the flickering images that appear on the screen of awareness—do this from the position of being your mind's best friend and letting it tell you how it secretly feels.

If the voices or stories become overwhelming, stop, relax, and see if you can just pay attention to the sounds you can hear in the room, then outside on the street, and then far away in the distance for a little while to regain the sense of spaciousness. The point isn't to get carried away by the details. It is to come out of the trance of your habitual storytelling and trust in the clarity of presence itself.

43

SENSING THE DIFFERENCE BETWEEN
KINDNESS AND SELF-HARM

Now that you've got a taste of what it is like to sense the stories your ego-mind is creating from the more primary position of your here-and-now awareness, you can begin to sense that broadly speaking, the stories about yourself fit into two categories: positive and negative. Real peace comes when we don't depend on either of these to define us and we find our home ground in the aliveness and clarity of presence itself. However, if you have the habit of getting caught in negative states, you will need to get to know them fully to understand why and how they arise and persist, before they begin to dissolve and give way to a deeper presence. A powerful and liberating way of viewing the kinds of stories about yourself that arise is asking the simple question "Is this kindness to myself, or is it self-harm?" This question is potent because it trains your attention to feel beneath the content of the story—the details, the reasons, the memories of situations, the "facts"—and simply feel what its energetic or heart quality is. Another way of putting it is "Does this story open me up or close me down?" This isn't an exercise in self-judgment, however (which is more of the same energy of self-harm) but rather an inquiry into what we actually are doing to ourselves in each present moment.

When I began looking at my mind through this lens, what I found was startling. I realized that most of the stories about "me" had a quality of violence to them. As the body became weaker and my ability to perform in the world became very limited, a default position of inner suspicion, a persistent mistrust of my own goodness, and a sense of being worthless became painfully apparent. The vulnerability, limitations, and helplessness that arose with continuous exhaustion, physical weakness, and an inability to think straight brought to light a fundamental bias in my mind and heart: "I am not a good enough person right now," "I am flawed, unworthy, useless." Throughout the day, many story lines, including the way I imagined I was being seen by "others" in my mind's eye, would come from and serve to reinforce this core feeling. In hindsight, however, it was a great opportunity to wake up to what had really been going on all my life—I had just been too busy resisting, denying, and distracting myself from it.

Before the body became ill, I had been a very driven person, always on the go, and always seeking to prove myself through achievements, creative pursuits, intellect—any way I could, to be honest. Yet there was always an underlying current of "not enough—gotta do more," and even when I was praised or appreciated, a core feeling of emptiness, deficiency, and lack persisted in the pit of my stomach. When I could muster the energy to prove myself in new ways, the feeling temporarily would get covered over. But at times when I couldn't, or when I was alone for too long, it would return.

In the first few years of my life as a Buddhist monk, these ego-based tendencies found a way to creep in and infiltrate my sense of self. It may sound strange to hear, given that the whole point of the lifestyle is to let go and "just be," but there I was, a young man in his twenties, trying to do everything he could to prove to his fellow monks that he was awesome. In fact, I tried to become the *best* monk by working the hardest, learning all the chanting the quickest, and being the most well-behaved—which ironically led to the other monks letting me know that they thought I was a bit too uptight. It was obvious to those who had been around a long time that my obsession with performance and competition was a compensation for an underlying tendency to judge myself and a loss of connection with my inner value. When it was suggested that I relax my "controlling tendencies,"

I recall thinking, "Yeah, yeah. I'll just continue the way I am, thanks." But when the body got sicker and the myriad ways of proving myself began to slip away, all of this changed.

I found myself immersed in a barrage of judgments and harsh internal voices telling me how I was failing, not measuring up, getting it all wrong. This was the first time in my life when I really had no option other than to face this habit of heart squarely. In the quiet of the afternoon, the spectral faces of my spiritual brothers would appear in my mind's eye, together with accompanying feelings of inadequacy related to particular tasks I had done that day, or more often, tasks that I *wasn't* able to do and self-images I wasn't able to live up to. I began to notice that the default position of my mind was to generate images and ideas of myself that were not based on kindness or compassion at all. For a period in my life, sitting with this tendency was like the movie *Groundhog Day*—like the same day was playing over and over—and the main star of the show was the voice of inner criticism, the tyrannical fault-finding mind, obsessed with concocting the feeling of "you're no good." Somewhere during this period I made what was a fascinating discovery: the mind didn't need an object or memory or anything based on reality at all to do this. Even on days when things had gone reasonably well and I had interacted with my friends lovingly and meaningfully, the mind would arise, like a snake from its den, with a subtle energetic quality that said, "Now, what can I feel wrong about today?" This was startling to see.

THE WISDOM OF SELF-KINDNESS

From the perspective of pure awareness that we have been inquiring into, even those deeply entrenched patterns and stories about being sick or chronically unwell, such as "I am flawed, broken, and useless," can be seen as creations of the ego-mind.

46

They arise in the present moment. They are constructed states
and not who we really are. Underneath them, we are always the
simple indefinable awareness and being that is here and now.

We will look into ways of directly connecting to and accessing this presence later in the book, but here I would like to invite
you to trust your own personal intuition of this dimension of
yourself. You can call it by any name—it doesn't matter. It is an
innocent habit that we have as humans to imagine that this truth
of being is somewhere outside of us—in an entity or a projected
ideal—but if not seen with wisdom, these projections can actually alienate ourselves from our true nature, which is what is
most intimate in this very moment. It is not in some other place
or some other time.

Allow yourself to feel that trust for a moment. Take it into
your heart of hearts. Relax into a sense of "Yeah, that's what's
true, I just keep forgetting it." Even if the experience of awareness itself is murky, hazy, or just a glimmer at the moment, that
is enough to show you that it's always here. It actually never left,
even though your attention did. Can you feel how kindness,
compassion, and benevolence are innate to this place in yourself? Can you sense how the moment you become unkind to
yourself you lose contact with the trust that you are whole, just
as you are, illness and all?

It is impossible to truly feel the blessings and benefits of this
wholeness if our mind and body are contracted through stories
and an energy of self-harm and inner violence. While the stories sometimes masquerade as a belief that if you punish or
criticize yourself, you will get better in "the future," what they
really do is cut you off from the source of true well-being, intelligence, and love in the present moment. Devoting yourself to
self-kindness is therefore an act of great wisdom. It turns your
compass around from the continuous feeling of wrongness, the
habitual resistance, and the sense that you are a "problem," to

ease, forgiveness, compassion, gentleness, and a connection to the completeness of simple presence itself.

THE EMBODIED EXPERIENCE OF KINDNESS

Now that you have a sense of the wisdom in relating to yourself, your body, and your illness with a heart of kindness, you can consciously explore, become curious, and remember what the quality of kindness, compassion, and love *feels* like in your own experience of being. There are many ways of approaching this, and their usefulness will depend on the resources of physical and mental energy you have available. Traditional meditations on self-kindness are often included in the framework of loving-kindness meditations and can involve a lot of mental energy. If you are exhausted or depleted, sometimes these can be counter-productive and leave you feeling more tired than when you began meditating. However, the principle is important—tuning in to and feeling for your innate capacity for openness, kindness, and love in the present moment.

When I say "innate," I am referring to the reality that this capacity is not something foreign to you. It is a natural part of our human nature, yet for most of us gets lost somewhere along the journey of life—usually in our childhood years. Because of real dangers, painful experiences, and our driven, competitive society, we learn to close our hearts and defend ourselves from being hurt. Many of us take this one step further and close our hearts to ourselves. When we become afraid of our own capacity for love and kindness, we begin to mistrust our own value in the process. After all, this quality of heart is often viewed as a weakness in our culture—and sadly we can even become hard-hearted toward ourselves, believing that this hardness is equivalent to strength.

In this journey you will discover that within kindness lies

the real strength. Far from being a form of weakness, it gives you access to a vital dimension of power and energy of spirit, of being, that can become a strength of commitment to loving yourself first and foremost. This isn't selfishness, by the way— this kind of relationship to ourselves automatically begins to radiate out to others. When kindness is aligned with wisdom and a real connection to presence, we recognize that we are all the same. This kindness belongs to *everyone*.

INVITING KINDNESS AND COMPASSION
BACK INTO YOUR HEART

When we are oriented toward presence itself, we sense that we, right here, this being sitting or lying here, are a living, breathing being—like all other living, breathing beings everywhere in the world. So how could we not deserve kindness and love? If we even have an inkling that any being, person, or creature is worthy of our love, then it naturally follows that we are too. Yet we often forget this, don't we? We forget how to offer ourselves the same love that often comes quite naturally toward others.

Stepping out of your story and coming into the directness of the moment will allow you to perceive your experience, your mind, your history, your strengths and weaknesses in this impersonal, objective way. This impersonal perspective doesn't make the heart cold and indifferent, though. It allows it to spontaneously come alive and resonate tenderly with what you find right here—this being you feel yourself to be, your difficulties, your struggle, the pain and discomfort present in your body. Attuning to awareness in this way creates a kind of deep intimacy with the present-moment experience of life—beginning right here with the totally unique experience of being you. And it invites your own loving heart to reveal itself, to come out of hiding.

You may want to pause now and feel if you can sense this

perspective—one that is both vast and spacious, the knowingness that we are a being like all others. One that invites you into a profound intimacy with yourself, touching the present moment, including all of your self-images and the stories of your life tenderly and directly with your awareness. Take as long as you like to remember this deeper perspective on your life.

When I started becoming conscious of this larger perspective, the first feeling I had was a kind of shock: "Why haven't I ever offered myself kindness?" "Why do I regard myself with so much harshness and judgment?" Sitting alone and reflecting on this, a feeling of deep sadness arose. As I stayed with it, relaxing the judgment and the cynical commentary that wanted to creep in, this feeling of sadness bloomed into what I would call a taste of universal compassion. Awareness began holding my very sense of myself, my life, and the difficulties I was experiencing in the resonant richness of this feeling, this deep intelligence. This wasn't sentimentality or self-pity, however—it was the first taste of the love that flows forth from deep in our being when we allow ourselves to be vulnerable. Paradoxically, this tenderness was accompanied by a feeling of energy and inner strength. I felt like I had come alive again. I felt like I had returned home.

The experience above was what I would call a *receptive* experience of the open heart and its expression as self-compassion. When our present-moment awareness is free from judgment and rests with the moment in a feeling of curiosity and real interest, we begin to intuit the possibility of receiving our body, our mind, and our situation with kindness and care. What arises is then met with a softness and warmth rather than a harsh or defended quality of heart.

It is also possible to engage in more *active* cultivation of caring, self-kindness, and expansiveness of heart. This involves deliberately summoning or calling forth the feeling itself through using memory, imagination, and a creativity of attention. The benefit of actively engaging in the process is that it retrains our heart, our being, to connect to the qualities of the open heart more spontaneously until they eventually become a natural way of relating to ourselves and those we encounter in our daily lives. Here I will offer a guided meditation to take you through one such process. It is important not to overthink what is being suggested—the real benefit will come from using the words on the page as reminders of your own capacity to feel the quality of warmth or connection in your own heart. Take time to get a sense of how to reconnect with these universal human qualities for yourself in your own unique way.

GUIDED MEDITATION:
REMEMBERING YOUR OWN LOVING NATURE

Settle back into the posture you find yourself in right now. Take some time to get comfortable, whether you are lying down reading this book or sitting upright. Make sure your belly and chest aren't folded in on themselves. See if you can allow them to be open and unguarded. Trust that right now there is no one you have to become, nothing you have to prove to yourself or anyone. There is nothing you have to defend yourself from. You are safe. You are free to be however you are.

If there are peripheral forces in your mind's eye that have the feeling tone of judgment, embarrassment, or mistrust, take a moment to acknowledge them and let them be. Right now these needn't concern you. They are just normal aspects of the human heart and mind. They are fine.

Resting in yourself in this way, feeling safe, and trusting in your own freedom to be as you are, see if you can connect to the intuitive dimension of heart underneath your thoughts and stories that are going on right now. This is the dimension that *feels,* that is moved by the beauty or sadness of life. Make a conscious decision now to come from that place for the next few minutes. Forget all the chatter of your thinking mind and place your attention more fully in this domain of heart-feeling.

Using your imagination and creativity, scan the depths of your memories of life so far for a moment when you felt love, kindness, or profound caring toward another person, animal, or as a response to life itself. The thinking mind is the tool you use to direct your attention, but the hub of it is your feeling awareness, your heart-sensitivity itself. Take some time to get a sense of what will work for you right now. If negative states or memories come up, just set them aside for now and stay focused on the theme of your search. Keep feeling and using your intuitive faculties as you revisit a moment in your life when you felt this love inside.

It may have been a dearly loved pet. For many of you it will resonate most strongly in the memory of an important person in your life you felt safe and trusting with—someone in whose presence you felt accepted, cared for, or regarded with affection. For some of you it may be a time alone in nature when you were a child, when you felt a feeling of freedom and joy for no reason and an inexplicable feeling of connection with all of life. Whichever of these feels most resonant for you from your own unique, personal memory bank, stay with it now. Use the mind to make the memory as rich as possible. See it in full color. Be there. Feel what you felt like. Take it in, again and again, as if you are sweeping over the scene to fill in the depth of your heart-feeling more fully each time.

Now that you are there, in your heart, become fully conscious of the well-being that is present in you. Notice how this well-being is connected, intimately, with your own capacity for love. Let that love touch you deeper. Let it flow from the inside out as you remember, with your whole body and mind, the experience you have chosen as your object of meditation.

Bathe in it. Delight in it.

Let it take you deeper into itself. Let it expand and fill you. Be bold with this heart-feeling. Make it vast. Let it open you. Dive into it. Now invite *yourself* into it. Gently hold out your heart to take in this being you feel yourself to be. Offer yourself this same loving, this same caring and compassion. Feel that your heart is wide enough to hold everything about yourself— your perceived faults, your illness and pain, your situation, and your history. All of it can be included in this field of resonant kindness.

Take your own time to stay with this feeling. Explore it for however long you like. If the mind gets distracted, starts to doubt, or becomes obsessed with "figuring it out," then just pause, relax, and come back to a sense that you are perfect just as you are right now. No judgment. Wherever you can open up a space that doesn't judge yourself for anything that arose—for how much or how little you were able to feel—that is the doorway of this loving itself. It is all just how it is.

Each time we go into this meditation, something new arises. Sometimes it is profound and takes us very deep. Other times it may just leave us wondering why we can't feel. Both are important, natural, and normal. Whatever arose for you is perfect in the unfolding of your own journey.

I should say here that kindness, compassion, and joy are all different expressions of the same quality of openheartedness that is our most natural being. When you are sick or in pain, you may often find that self-compassion is the expression that comes most easily, as it is love's response to suffering. It can also come through gratitude for the web of interconnection that supports you, as we will see later, or from a sudden waking up to the importance of living from kindness itself. But regardless of how this warmth arises, all of these qualities have the same characteristics: an open, soft transparency, a radiance and vitality of presence, and perhaps most important when we are sick, the absence of self-judgment and a contracted state of being.

When we sense the beauty and deep relief of self-kindness, compassion, and caring—and how much freer life feels when we live from these qualities—the contracted heart sticks out like a sore thumb. We realize that the doorway to true well-being always lies within the open heart, and never through any form of inner violence. In our being we begin to sense directly that self-criticism, judgment, and shame about being ill don't feel well at all. In fact, they create the most painful and crippling form of human illness—illness of being. The symptoms of this illness are feelings of alienation and a lack of happiness, a lack of contentment and joy. We lose the capacity to meet ourselves with compassion and love. Losing our health, our job, or our abilities are all devastating forms of loss, but this is the greatest loss there is.

4

Equanimity: The Strength Hidden in Openness

NOW THAT YOU have a sense of your own capacity for self-kindness and a whole body and mind approach to awareness and presence, it is time to explore how the two come together in a pragmatic way. As we have seen, one of the main obstacles to inner well-being that arises when our body is sick, in pain, or experiencing ongoing exhaustion is our ingrained habit of resistance and the myriad ways we reject our present-moment experience. In order to counter and transform these habits, we need to cultivate a deeper strength. The experience of *samadhi,* the whole-body and mind unification in presence, provides a foundation for this to emerge in a way that can permeate all aspects of our life, not just quiet experiences in meditation. When our experience of life is physically challenging, painful, and limited, recognizing this capacity is nothing short of life-changing. In Buddhist texts, this quality of strength in presence is referred to as *equanimity.* While this English translation of the Pali word *upekkha* can conjure up images of indifference or cold aloofness, the actual experience is quite the opposite.

For us in the West it is common to associate strength with hardness. Our cultural mythology around strength can be seen in the protagonists of action movies, superheroes, or police dramas, where the main character is tough, rarely expresses emotion, and yet is unaffected by grave danger, pain, or difficulty. This ideal can seem very appealing—we would all love to be invincible, unwavering in the face of challenges, and unflappable. Indeed, these qualities are desirable and bear some resemblance to the spiritual dimension of being that can be cultivated through meditative inquiry. However, when it comes to relating to ourselves, our bodies, and our own pain, the shadow side of emulating this kind of ideal can often be an inner hardening against our present-moment experience. As we have seen, when we relate to physical illness and pain in this way, the results can be a worsening of symptoms and an increase of the sense of being divided inside. This sense of inner division then gives power to perceptions of illness being wrong and stories about the future that perpetuate a state of anxiety and fear just below the surface.

Yet we need inner strength when we live with chronic illness. Rather than being walled off, hard, and unfeeling, this kind of strength is in fact the opposite—it is the capacity to be present for both the unpleasantness of experience and the pleasure, joys, and highs, with a sense of being grounded in the present moment, in awareness itself. An equanimous heart comes about through standing firm in the midst of experience while remaining open, receptive, and sensitive at the same time. This is the difference between true strength of presence and the idealized version we see in the media. On the surface of it, qualities like receptivity and sensitivity can appear as expressions of weakness, but this is only true if they overwhelm us from the ego position and collapse the mind into the turbulence of stories about ourselves, the past, and the future. When combined with a here-and-now embodied awareness, however, these qualities become gateways to the direct experience of inner strength and a confidence in the indestructible nature of our deepest presence itself.

OPENNESS IS COURAGE

While hardening, defending, and pushing through life is a kind of strength, it lacks the quality that forges true inner strength—courage. For most of us, it is more appealing to go out and conquer the world, shelve or deny our true feelings, and live in a constant state of restless activity than to actually feel what it feels like to just be alive. Why is it so hard to be open to what is here right now?

Often the feeling we are afraid of contacting is just the residual unpleasantness built up in our system through habitual distraction and outward seeking. There is a layer of discomfort that lurks under the surface of our constant search for the next thing that—if we are honest—we really don't want to feel. In fact, when we are presented with the option of meeting it in openness we may realize that we are actually afraid of it. When what is waiting here for us is illness and pain, this fear can get very strong, so we need to meet it wisely and with sensitivity.

The first step in unfolding this fear of openness is recognizing that your presence can be here for all conditions. When you are grounded in the wisdom that knows stories of yourself, the past, or the future as fabrications that you are creating in this very moment, you are always safe. The itchiness and irritability of the present moment is just that—it feels uncomfortable, yes, but your presence remains awake and aware. This act of opening into the actual feeling of the body and mind in the present moment is therefore an act of great courage. It isn't the grandiose act of a superhero, but it is a subtle kind of everyday courage that makes you strong inside. This is the heart of equanimity.

Training oneself in this kind of undefended receptivity to the present moment is a process of trial and error. In fact, it is a lifetime's work. When we enter into the process, we find that our awareness swings between either being caught in the stories that underlying patterns of energy spawn or spacing out into a state of dissociation and numbness. This isn't wrong—these are just the two default positions of the human mind. Through this process we gradually come to know for ourselves what is sometimes called the Middle Way. It is the way in between those two default positions of being caught in the whirlwind of fragmented mind states and freezing up by dissociating. It is the way of fully feeling what is here without grabbing on to it or pushing it down. It is both the knowingness that can see "Ah, I'm making up a whole bunch of stuff about the future, who I am in the present moment, or what these feelings mean about my life" and the receptive sensitivity that can feel *how* those states feel in the body—in the gut, the chest, the belly, the shoulders, or the face. The act of engaging in the process is what gradually reveals the underlying quality of equanimity in itself. It is a stillness that doesn't need to react against what we find right here and now in our body and mind. This stillness isn't dead and cold, however. If we remain connected to the life force driving our thinking mind—the fear, worry, or anger—this very life force transforms into an aliveness of presence. You could say that this turbulent energy gives itself back to presence when we meet it without repression or clinging—but with a receptive awareness instead. The sense of stillness becomes more vital, energetic, and potent the more we remain connected to how we actually feel being here in this moment. When the stillness of presence is energized in this way, it becomes an inner strength that stays with us, even when we are not engaged in any formal practice. It brings us back home, out from the fragmented realm of mental images and ideas, into a centered, grounded awareness that is open to life and strong enough to meet it without reacting, judging, or collapsing.

BALANCING THE MASCULINE AND FEMININE

As we have seen, equanimity can often be framed up primarily in terms of what I would call a more masculine archetype—rigidity, hardness, solidity—which leaves us lacking in more of the feminine principles of openness, receptivity, and the capacity to be intimate with experience. Of course, these are very broad ways of talking about the masculine and feminine principles, but I have found this framework useful when exploring the actual experience of equanimity in relation to discomfort, pain, and fatigue in the body. Whenever I tighten, harden, or defend against an experience of exhaustion, for example, the life force of the body begins to feel more depleted. The very act of closing off awareness from the here-and-now experience in turn shuts off whatever reserves of energy are left in the bodily system. The subjective experience becomes more fraught, and my mind gets hooked into a particular narrative of negativity, such as "Why am I so tired?" or "Oh, come on, stupid body. Not this again?" Do these sound familiar? You probably know them well! As we have seen earlier, this experience of ill will, if pursued through repetitive habit, can turn into a mode of hating the body, which has devastating effects.

So here we can see the relationship between the here-and-now experience of hardening against experience and ensuing states of negativity, ill will, and hatred. Yet we often take this stance because the opposite seems worse—becoming depressed and impotent or drowning in murky states of fear and despair.

Hardening against our experience feels like the noble thing to do, and in a way there is a strength that we are generating in the mind in order to do this. So as with all that we find in our experience, there is no need to judge it. The art is to distill the quality of strength from its shadow of blocking out, dissociating from, or repressing the here-and-now experience of body and mind. In order to do this, we need to be willing to fail a little, to lose some of our apparent control on conditions. The magic, however, is that if we do this in full presence rather than unconsciously falling into a state of weakness, there is a new kind of harmonization that occurs—we discover that we don't need to control in the way we thought we did, and that in relinquishing the death grip on the present moment, we don't lose our strength at all. We gain it.

The strength that is gained through relaxing the apparent control that comes from inner hardening is the strength of presence itself. It is different from the strength of ego, which always has a walled-off feeling to it—inside it we feel as if we are encased in a hermetically sealed armor of "me." When this armor of "me" solidifies, anything that is seen as a threat to its survival, such as illness or pain, becomes an enemy. The strength of presence is something of an altogether different nature. Although vulnerability destabilizes ego strength, when it is held with wisdom, it also empowers the strength of presence.

Equanimity is a very powerful quality to bring into our everyday experience of living with chronic illness, because it generates a trust that we can open to what is here, right now, with interest in feeling the actual experience of being alive. A lifetime of habitual yet subconscious fear is released in the process. Living without this fear is the real strength that becomes possible. Within the strength that can be present for the mess of life—the failures, loss, pain, and limitations that come with illness—we rediscover real meaning, real value. Standing firm in an open, sensitive presence opens us up to resources of joy and well-being at the core of our being itself. We realize that we are always right here, despite how the body feels and what the mind is telling us. The feeling of "here-ness" gathers a momentum into itself and blossoms into a heart-feeling of freedom. This freedom knows that everything is OK. It's all just as it is.

NONREACTIVITY

In order to taste this balance of steadfastness and vulnerability for yourself, you will need to look at one of its main obstacles: reactivity. When you allow yourself to feel exactly how you are feeling in this moment, you may notice a knee-jerk reaction that very quickly takes you into a thought, a story, or a perception of what the feeling means. Can you notice that tendency in yourself? It often happens with lightning speed, and you can find yourself lost in planning your grocery shopping for tomorrow or ruminating about who you are and what you did to make yourself so ill. If you find this happening, then you can be very sure there was a moment of unseen reactivity in relation to what you encountered in your here-and-now feeling awareness.

Reactivity is what diminishes the power and strength of presence. Presence is lost in that moment. Of course, sometimes the feelings you encounter will be beyond your threshold of what you can feel, particularly in the case of acute pain, so if this is the case, it may be more beneficial to focus on self-kindness and creating a space of compassion for yourself instead. However, instead of doing this through habitual reactivity, see if you can make this choice consciously and through trusting that you know what this moment needs. Remember that you are free to choose how to attend to this moment. Remembering this takes the power away from reactivity and places it back in the hub of your present-moment awareness. I say this here so that you feel your freedom in this moment. Only you know what you need right now—sometimes it is just a quiet space of relaxed, loving attention, while at other times you may feel clear and well-resourced enough to play the edges of your here-and-now presence in a way that can meet and hold the reactive mind. The choice is always your own. You can never go wrong with kindness.

If you are feeling like there is enough clarity and energy in your mind to explore this further, ask yourself right now, "What is it like to be fully sensitive to this moment without reacting against it and without making a story about it?" Take a moment to feel that for yourself.

If your mind feels like it is all over the place, messy, broken, or dejected, what is it like to be fully present for that very stuff? No reaction. No resistance. Just relax into presence alongside whatever is here. There is no need to judge it or give extra meaning to it by feeling that you are failing, unspiritual, not-good-at-this-awareness-stuff, or anything at all. Remain connected to a quality of great kindness and generosity toward yourself.

Where do you feel reactivity in the body? Can you sense an energy that arises to deflect, detract, or push attention away as you get nearer an uncomfortable feeling in the body, a painful emotion, or a mind state that feels out of control, like it might take you over perhaps? What is it like to relax that energetic impulse and stand firm in awareness itself? This doesn't mean getting lost in what you encounter—it is that poise, right in the middle, when you are neither repressing nor clinging to what you find. Whatever the conditions of body and mind, they are all just the scenery of this moment. You can rest in the presence that is always free from identification with it.

MEDITATION ON EQUANIMITY

Imagine yourself as a mighty tree rooted in the middle of a fast-moving river. The currents beat up against it, eddy around it, spray it with water, but the tree remains firm. Its roots go deep underground. The tree doesn't try to stop the flow of the river. How could it? The river is just the river. But it stands firm. It feels the river against it, ever changing, ever flowing, but it is unwavering. Can you feel what it would be like to be that tree right now? Your mind, your feelings, and the state of your body are the river. Your aware presence, the receptive knowingness at the heart of your being, is the tree. Let the mind be the mind, as messy, dark, or confused as it is. No problem. Hold it with great kindness. Let the body be as it is, as weak, painful, or exhausted. It is just this way. It is not your fault. Please don't follow those thoughts. The condition of your body too is like the flowing river. It just flows. And in all of this your presence can stand firm, extending its roots deeper into the open ground of presence itself, rather than making anything out of what you find here and now in your body, your thoughts, your inner voice, or your emotions. Rest here and now—vulnerable yet standing firm. This is equanimity.

BEING HERE, FOR THIS

Very often in my own life, this sense of the strength in presence has arisen when I have been very ill. I remember a period during my time living as a monk when the energy levels of the body were so low that it just wasn't possible to even make it through one meditation session without collapsing. It wasn't as if we were sitting all day, either, and I frequently missed the morning meditations. This was the one meditation session I had to attend in a given day. At times my body was so depleted and drained that there was no option but to very quietly walk out of the meditation hall and into the adjoining "monks' room" where we stored our few belongings. Still clad in formal robes and so wiped out that even walking was an arduous experience, I would lie down on my back and just be there—the "collapsed monk." I say it with some humor, as even though the experience was humiliating for the ego-mind, the whole situation was quite ridiculous. I still remember it with a smile on my face, despite how weak and fragile my physical system had become.

As I lay there, I would begin to notice the surface layer of the present moment—a momentum of stories washing through the mind's eye—stories of failure, dejection, and not-being-good-enough. "Here I go again . . ." the inner voice would say, often mirrored by projected images of what I imagined the others in the meditation hall were thinking. "He's lazy," "You give up too easily," "You should try harder"—phrases such as these accompanied the images as ways of attacking my choice to relinquish control and instead just rest. So I would just slow down and notice, "Ah, here are the judgments again, right on time." Seeing this flow of habitual self-criticism for what it was opened up a deeper space in the heart and mind to just be with the body. Lying down was actually very helpful for enabling me to feel the exact experience of what was in the moment without hardening against it or being pushed out into painful narratives about my life. Choosing the option of self-kindness and establishing that as the primary attitude allowed me to remain in tune with what the moment needed. As I relaxed the identification with stories of self-judgment, a feeling of "rightness" filled my heart. I was being here, for *this,* in the way that it needed, as opposed to the way that would please my self-image, which had already taken a battering.

The feeling of relaxed but present "rightness" allowed awareness to remain steady with the realm of bodily feeling. The textures, tones, and sensations of bodily experience became more palpable as presence relaxed out of the reactivity and self-criticism. As the story of "me" receded into the background of awareness, it began to feel as if presence was filling me up with itself. What had been experienced as a void, an emptiness, a lack, was becoming flooded with a powerful sense of awareness and light. The more the heart remained open, vulnerable, and steady in the present-moment field of sensation, the more this awareness consumed the experience. The sensations themselves—feelings of weakness, fatigue, and discomfort—lost the negative meaning I habitually ascribed them, and curiously, the whole body began to feel as if it *was* presence itself. This experience was accompanied by a feeling of well-being that wasn't euphoric or excited (the thinking mind remained exhausted, with a head-ache, and weak)—but rather a quiet trust that the present moment is absolutely fine. Though I felt myself in a state of naked vulnerability lying there in my formal robes, unable to sit up, prove anything, or "look the part," the mind was steadfast in its presence and sensitive to the whole experience of the moment. This stillness, the relaxing of reactivity, revealed an underlying dimension of mind, heart, and being that could directly taste its own fullness simply by being it. Words don't capture it very well; they can only point to the direct, personal experience.

Soon I would hear the bell ring in the meditation hall and I would shuffle myself back into a seated slump. There would be a sudden whoosh of exhaustion and dizziness that returned as I reengaged a more everyday mode of consciousness, but the feeling of equanimity remained. I recognized that if I had continued trying to push through the body and forced myself to sit up straight, the result would not have been equanimity but rather a tight and contracted state, and the mind and body not only would have been exhausted but angry and irritable as well. It was a very powerful example of how being receptive and vulnerable to experience can actually bring forth great power in the mind, and one that significantly shaped the way I relate to fatigue and exhaustion ever since.

5

Meeting the Dark Emotions

WHEN YOU LIVE with the ongoing experience of illness, pain, and limitation, you aren't going to be happy all the time. This is the reality, isn't it? Yet it doesn't mean something is going wrong. It is the natural response to painful physical feeling, frustrated desire, and the loss of familiar ways of being and performing in the world. The blessing and the curse of chronic illness is that it reveals a whole other side to life, one that you may have suppressed or tried to wall off from your awareness in the past—the shadow side of the human mind. This realm of turbulent emotions such as fear, despair, anger, or grief doesn't need to be judged as "bad," nor does it mean we are failing. On the contrary, being prepared to meet these forces of mind and heart squarely and with a quality of creative self-compassion is a process of becoming fully human and allowing our capacity for presence to open, deepen, and unfold into an intimacy with who and how we are. It is an invitation into the real transformation that comes about not through repression, becoming someone else, or clinging to an ideal of who we should be, but through applying wisdom and a compassionate awareness to the facts of the human heart, just as they are.

Allowing ourselves to deeply feel our inner life with kindness and equanimity and to become consciously vulnerable in the face of dark or difficult emotions doesn't mean believing them or acting them out. This process relies once again upon the Middle Way—between trying to harden against and defend ourselves from certain feelings, on the one hand, and getting absorbed in their energy and stories on the other. This is the way of here-and-now awareness. It is a dynamic response to each moment, each situation as it is presenting itself in the immediacy of the present moment. Sometimes, as you will see, you need to engage your mind's stories to catalyze a conscious connection to the currents of energy and emotion that lie beneath the realm of images and ideas, while at other times, when these forces are persistent and powerful, all you need to do is come out of the head and bring presence to the sensations in the body. Both methods of applying your attention require the qualities of heartfelt self-kindness and steadfast presence that you have already been exploring in yourself.

If this way of conscious vulnerability with the dark, wayward, or negative energies of heart is completely new to you, it may be useful to focus more on letting go of self-judgment and bringing kindness and clarity to the whole perspective you have on your situation first. The prospect of meeting strong energies in the heart and mind can seem overwhelming or bring up a feeling of "Not another thing I have to deal with." If that is the case, then for now I would recommend you skip the rest of this chapter and continue reading—until you feel the call to revisit it. As with all aspects of this work of inquiry and presence, you yourself are the one who knows the right time for a practice or a way of looking. There are no "shoulds." Trust your own sense of what is right for you at this time with your unique body and

mind. Sometimes just putting your hand on your heart and re-
minding yourself "I am OK" is an entire universe of relief that
needs nothing added to it.

Indeed, from the perspective of our true presence, we are already perfect in this moment, just as we are. The art of allowing
turbulent, dark, and messy emotions to be held in a space of
compassionate presence is not intended to be a project to fix or
get rid of anything. Instead, it is another way of using the raw
material of ongoing illness or pain as a vehicle for transformation and well-being rather than for solidifying feelings of failure
or defeat. Most of you will have experienced some form of up-
welling turbulence or downward moving darkness during the
course of your illness. This is normal. At some point you will
notice that, along with ways of bringing brightness and a positive
outlook to your situation, there is also a call to relinquish the
habit of blocking or denying the shadow side of your heart and to
be courageous enough to meet it with vulnerability and awareness. This call comes from a deep source of wisdom in yourself.
It knows that the treasures contained within the real are far more
exquisite and precious than those that our mind can construct
through will or imagination. Perhaps it also trusts that through
vulnerability and steadfast presence we won't be destroyed or
overwhelmed—we will instead come back to life with freshness,
wholeness, and a newfound sense of aliveness. From my own
experience and from working with others in similar situations,
this trust is well founded.

SUSTAINABLE WELL-BEING

Right now you may be wondering, "Why would I want to feel the
negative stuff, anyway? Why not just be happy?" This is a fair
question, and of course, happiness and well-being are preferable
to their opposite. There is no need to seek out more misery in the

midst of a situation that is already challenging. However, this invitation to open to the drives and currents of turbulence that afflict the mind is actually a call to feel inner well-being in a far deeper and more sustainable way than you may be used to. Although we all want to be happy, the more we grasp it, the more elusive it becomes. Our lives can end up feeling like a roller-coaster ride where we long for the ups and fear or resent the downs. Living with illness highlights this tendency in very stark ways. Because of the loss of control, diminished energy, and weakening of our life force, we begin to become very aware of the fragile nature of all constructed mind states. We recognize that the happiness we have been used to is highly dependent on conditions that could change at any time—if we eat the wrong food, if the weather changes, if we have a sleepless night, or if we have one of our "bad days" on the level of physical functioning. If happiness is dependent upon those conditions going the way we want them to, we can end up feeling like life is a continuous battle, with a few victories amid an ocean of failure. Trying to force ourselves to be happy when we can't digest food, have a piercing migraine, or barely have enough energy to walk can quickly become another form of violence toward ourselves. We are subconsciously saying, "I don't want to feel bad. I won't allow it." There is only so long we can grit our teeth in this way. Sooner or later, a deeper surrender is required.

Meeting the edge of this surrender requires sensitivity, readiness, and alert awareness, however. It cannot be forced, and can only happen with a heart of kindness and generosity toward ourselves just as we are. As we explore two significant areas of emotional turbulence that arise in the context of living with chronic illness or pain, we will encounter a basic underlying principle that applies to awareness practice: the act of trusting in the refuge of presence itself opens the doorway to transformation. From the perspective of here-and-now awareness, this framework is of key importance when working with painful and agitated emotions. It rests upon the understanding that our presence itself is enhanced, deepened, and revitalized whenever we meet currents of emotion in the body *just as they are,* with an open, curious attention. This meeting of the here-and-now experience has a different flavor from merely indulging its apparent reality, however. It requires a shift from being identified with the worlds and the stories that strong emotions spawn to being the ground of your innate presence itself, seeing stories as stories and knowing that all ideas about "my past" or "my future" are selective, subjective perceptions, arising in this very moment. Orienting oneself to the ground of presence is not a dissociative process either. As we have explored in the previous chapter, it is the same feeling of being like a mighty tree rooted in the middle of a fast-moving river. In this case, however, it is the very drives and currents of our human-ness that we are being present for.

FEAR AND DESPAIR

Living with illness can be terrifying. Any degree of loss of control, limitation, and the inability to function opens us to previously unmet fear. This is just the way our human mind works. When this loss of control persists, we may find that it becomes hard to appear calm and upbeat like we have been used to. We can feel like an undertow of fear is beginning to infiltrate our familiar mode of existence. Sometimes it is like a vortex or a black hole wanting to pull our mood downward, while at other times it can be more like being in a tiny boat, buffeted around by enormous waves in the middle of a dark ocean storm. Fear is a natural part of our heart and mind, however, and need not be judged. It can be a very useful energy when it is in the service of wisdom, such as when it serves our intuition to make or not make a decision. Think of the fear that arises before you say or do something you know will be harmful to yourself or others, for example. This is a kind of wise fear that acts as a touchstone and a guide and ceases soon after it has arisen. The fear we are looking at here is something of a different nature, however. It is the existential fear that constellates around stories of "me" and "my life," and becomes entranced by fabrications of a future time, whether it be later today, next week, or twenty years from now. It wants everything to be OK yet instinctively feels that this OK-ness will come about through contracting, closing, and worrying, through generating the causes for *un-OK-ness* in the heart.

When we see that this activity of mind is the very cause of the deepest kind of distress and existential suffering that could arise in the future—our own disconnection from true safety, the ground of peace and wholeness in the heart—we can begin to transform our relationship to fear. When we don't, fear erodes and undermines both the potential for feeling a sense of inner safety and trust and the precious resources of vitality and creativity that allow for a wise responsiveness to the conditions of life.

THE FEAR OF FEAR

For many of you there may be a preliminary stage in this process of exploration: whenever you feel an inkling that fear may be at work, a secondary fear of the fear itself arises, which then freezes your emotional being. Notice if that is the case for you. This is completely natural. You just may need to pause and reflect for a moment. What connotations does the idea of experiencing fear, consciously, in full presence, bring up for you? Does it feel welcome or unappealing? Do you feel like you can be present for it or is there a current of energy that arises in your belly or your chest that says "No"? If there is, just pause now and get curious about it. What, really, are you saying "no" to? What qualities of

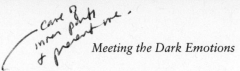
your own heart and mind could you trust in in order for that "no" to soften?

Softening that response is a very powerful starting point. It is in many ways the doorway to any kind of inner well-being you will experience. Of course it is easier to say "yes" to the pleasant aspects of life and of your psyche, isn't it? This work does require commitment and persistence—coming up against the "no" response again and again and feeling for yourself how much you can soften, open, and trust in the strength of presence itself. In this process you will also realize for yourself that nothing is destroyed in the process; in fact, everything comes back to life. But this knowledge needs to be your own and to unfold in your own time, through your own direct experience of courageously experimenting with new ways of being.

For myself, beginning to soften this fear of fear was a profound revelation. I realized that while I thought this habit was protecting me, it was actually giving power to subterranean patterns of fearfulness. When the energy and power of fear is locked up inside of our system, it secretly has a mind of its own. It can paralyze our capacity for emotional intelligence, creativity, and openness. It erodes our inner resources of self-kindness and compassion and generates a momentum of "I can't trust life." When we feel we can't trust life, the mirror image of that perception comes back to us one hundred and eighty degrees: we consequently feel "I can't trust myself." We *are* life. In my own journey, recognizing that the fear of fear is actually a fear of *myself* has been the key piece of the puzzle. I realized that I was actually afraid of falling apart, of not being able to hold it all together. Within these ideas was a deeper underlying fear: I was afraid of just being myself.

From the position of the ego-mind, habitually grasping an image of who we should be—strong, competent, helpful, giving, above-all-this, winning, for example—the imperfect reality and vulnerability of our human hearts and minds, just as they are, appears threatening and forbidden. When our bodies become ill and our energy levels start to wane, the habit of clinging to such fixed ideas is seen for the pain it actually is. However, the beautiful paradox is that the more we actually allow ourselves to feel how we are feeling, turbulence and all, the more our real potential for manifesting the qualities of heart we really long for shines forth—it is only through being real that the deeper treasures of our human being reveal themselves. It is only through opening to the darkness that we can become the light.

QUESTIONING THE STORIES OF FEAR

Very often we don't notice that fear is actually the underlying force driving our patterns of thought and ways of perceiving ourselves. Instead we are caught in certain kinds of stories about the future and preoccupied with thinking even more thoughts about those thoughts themselves. The power of inquiring in this way of direct, embodied awareness is that we can begin to unpack and unfold the very fabric of these stories themselves and develop a familiarity with them that allows us to notice them for what they are more quickly in the future. It can take a while to recognize, "Oh, this is fear." The stories the mind spins around fear can seem absolutely real—we view the scenarios we are fixated on as actual facts rather than thoughts that are arising in this very moment, whether they are based around thoughts of not being able to cope in the future, desolate scenarios of being abandoned and penniless, or fixed ideas of whether or how our health is going to decline.

However, in reality we don't know. Some of our guessing may prove to have a correlation to a future reality, but on the most basic level, right now, we actually don't know. Take that in for a moment. Can you sense the fundamental reality that this is pointing to? As has always been the case, events and conditions flow in ways our mind never could have imagined.

Allow yourself to pause and reflect on the significance of this truth. What would it be like to admit this fundamental fact to yourself right now? Is there a sense of relief and refreshment that returns to the feeling of being here right now in your body? Or is there another layer of fear around uncertainty itself? If there is, just pause and breathe, connecting to your body, and hold it gently. I would like to suggest that there is nothing to fear in uncertainty—in fact, it is the gateway to a real sense of fullness and trust in the heart, on account of the fact that it is actually true. In many ways it is the *only* certainty. Letting that fresh breeze into the heart, in the present moment, empties out all the mind-made shadows clouding awareness. Knowing you don't know, and allowing the mind to rest in that knowing, is a powerful and peaceful state of being.

This doesn't mean feeding the energy of doubt, however. We are not saying to ourselves, "I don't know, but I have to figure it out." That is knowing we don't know but hating the fact! This kind of doubt, the compulsive kind that won't let your mind rest, also needs to be met with the strength and clarity of equanimity and wisdom. As with all mind states, the question to ask is "Does this open me up to well-being in the present moment, or does it drag me down into more fear and worry?" Compulsive doubt leads to the latter. Can you sense that for yourself? As well as knowing we don't know, we can also know the energy of doubt directly, clearly, and spaciously as a present-moment phenomenon. Feeling for the current of sensation underneath the details of the storytelling mind, such as "Will it?" "But what if?" "Am I?" and opening up the space of awareness to know, penetratingly and directly, *"Ahhh . . . this is doubt!"* is the key. It is doubt. Feel doubt as doubt. How does doubt feel? Pull a face to give expression to it. Make it come alive in full awareness. It

doubt

is a close relative of fear and anxiety but often hides as an un-seen link in the causal process of mental suffering and affliction. To bring it into the light in this way is very empowering. I often find myself asking the mind, "What's that you say? *Ahhh,* hello doubt. How do you feel?" Doubt then lets me know how it feels, directly and viscerally, rather than taking me into a plethora of conflicting and unresolved speculations about the present moment, the past, or the future. When it comes to the future, doubt is especially cunning at co-opting our present moment mind state and taking us into stories—what better food for doubt could there be than something that hasn't happened yet? So patiently and compassionately meeting it *as* itself, rather than being caught in its self-perpetuating (and thus agitating and depleting) agenda, is where our real power lies.

However, as we have seen, there is another kind of doubt that is of great benefit. This isn't the compulsive kind that drags us into speculation but rather the Great Doubt that is spoken of in the Zen tradition. This doubt is aligned with wisdom and presence and is an act of choice rather than an unconscious habit. Doubting a future that appears to be absolutely true, in this case, is that which allows us to acknowledge the uncertainty of our mind's projections and starve the energy of fear of its food and sustenance. This kind of doubt opens up a space in awareness that glimpses the emptiness of the present moment. This emptiness is the wholeness and relaxation that unfolds when the complicated, conflicting, and ultimately groundless matrix of future thinking dissolves. The feeling is one of homecoming and relief.

So the pragmatism of really taking the truth of uncertainty into our heart lies in its power to bring to light the transparency and unreality of our fixed ideas of what will happen—later today, this year, or in the distant future. Taking it into the heart is an act of radically waking up. We wake up out of the realm of half truths, speculation, and mental fog, into the crystal clear aliveness of presence itself. From this place we can begin to meet the energy of worry or anxiety that has been driving our stories in an empowered way rather than merely feeling like we are being washed away or engulfed by a river of fear. When there is clarity around the nature of the mind's stories and a trust that the underlying reality is in fact uncertainty itself, the feeling-presence of equanimity returns to our heart. As we have seen, this isn't a repressive force but rather the strength of being able to stand firm in the midst of the primal currents of being without being dragged under or pulled over the rapids. From this vantage point in the heart, fear can be met as it is—an energetic movement of mind, felt in and through the body right now.

When my health was at its worst, working with fear was a daily challenge. In fact, for a certain amount of time, my mind was unconsciously busy working away at strengthening fear rather than understanding or unfolding it. As the stomach's motility (and therefore capacity to digest food) became increasingly limited and the energy levels of the body began dropping significantly as a result, a powerful and compelling current of fear began to take hold. This wasn't the fear of wearing the wrong kind of clothes to work or of having said the wrong thing to a friend over coffee—it was and is deep stuff, as I am sure many of you know intimately. However, in the process, the thinking mind had co-opted the natural energy of fear itself and turned it into fixed, encrusted notions of "my life," usually involving a projection in time of about ten to fifteen years. The projection wasn't pretty. It was miserable. Along the way I had begun, subconsciously, to believe that this reality was certain—it was a fact, and that's just the way it was going to be. This belief in a fixed future weighed heavily on the heart and eventually bubbled up as panic attacks in the middle of the afternoon, right after an hour-long nap. The feeling that arose viscerally in the body was one of dread, terror, and darkness. My heart would begin to race and the thoughts in the mind would go headlong into disaster scenarios. This intensity continued for a few weeks, until one afternoon.

Having fallen asleep in a post-meal slump, I woke up with a start to this now familiar feeling of dread and terror in the pit of my stomach. It is hard to describe in words, but it felt all-encompassing and filled the entire experience of the present moment. Even though I was nestled in a hut in a Buddhist monastery surrounded by tranquil forest sounds, everything I saw or heard was filtered with this feeling. The sound of the raven, the breeze rustling through the trees—everything. Sitting upright, awareness began to ask, "What *is* this?" The nightmarish nature of this state had become so agonizing that presence summoned the energy to face it squarely and courageously for the first time in years. The mind, suddenly energized with determination and penetrating clarity, felt for the real answer. I found myself asking, "Why am I doing this?" and "What is this, *really*?"

It was only then that awareness encountered layers of stories that had become so familiar, so everyday, that I had forgotten that the mind itself made them up. As awareness looked into these stories, it dawned on me: none of it was true. It was as if attention had been so sucked into this stream of future-oriented thinking that it had forgotten to return to the reality of the present. But I suddenly remembered, "This is all made up. None of these stories are certain. I have no idea what's going to happen next week, let alone ten years from now." In that moment the intensity of the fear abated and presence returned, refreshing, energized, and clear—as if I had actually woken up out of a dream. And I heard the mind say, "Don't believe that stuff." It was a very significant moment. While the undercurrents of fear didn't just disappear immediately, meeting them *as* fear for the first time opened up a space of inner strength and clarity that could begin to feel the present moment arising, moving, rippling, and sinking of fear, without solidifying it into a fixed view of "my life." Looking back on that time, ten years ago, it is now so clear that those projections were mere fantasy. The disastrous life I imagined would unfold, including the absolute certainty of my health getting worse, proved to be a mental fabrication. It arose in the present moment back then. That's the only place it ever existed. It is marvelous and breathtaking to really take that into the heart.

When you are weak and depleted, it takes all the strength you have to challenge the flow of mind energy that has been kidnapped by fear and despair. But even seeing the stories *as* stories for a few minutes, clearly and directly, can transform your relationship to the arising of fear itself.

FEELING FEAR IN THE BODY

Now that you have some tools to explore and deconstruct the stories of your own fear that arise in relation to the experience of illness, it is time to go to the heart of the matter: the present-moment experience of fear in the body. While it is indeed powerful to see through the apparent reality that stories of fear conjure up in the mind's eye, it is equally powerful to develop the capacity to meet the feeling of fear in the immediacy of embodied presence itself. In the light of nonjudgmental awareness, self-acceptance, and the steadfastness of equanimity, the question changes from "How can I get rid of this fear?" to "What is fear anyway?"

Asking this question is not an analytical search for answers on the level of the cognitive mind but rather a curious exploration of the actual feeling quality of fear—the textures, movements, physical effects, and associated sensations—that are manifesting in the present moment. What does it do to your shoulders or your throat? How does it feel in the belly and the right or left side of the torso? Does it creep into the muscles of your face? Can you feel it in your arms? What can you feel around your chest? How does the overall sensation of your body feel when fear is present? Does it become heavy, like a burden you have to carry around? Or do you lose contact with it and feel as if your body has disappeared altogether?

 As we will see with other kinds of turbulent, dark emotions, sometimes it is necessary to reengage a fear story in order to regain access to the direct embodied experience underneath. However, it is important not to skip the first step of seeing into the fabricated nature of any thought about the future. As we have seen above, it is essential to develop this objective, crystal-clear knowing of the make-believe nature of stories before we can hold them in a way that allows us to access the here-and-now sensations of the underlying energy itself. I mention this here because a very common experience for folks beginning this exploration is a kind of duality of "I'm either totally *in* it or I can't feel anything at all." It is a natural experience to move from complete absorption in the state of fear to a kind of dissociation where the energy has been blocked out or walled off from awareness. In this practice we are clearing a pathway in between those two default positions so that we can touch the heart of the experience clearly, compassionately, and with transformative wisdom.

It is possible to rest in the strength of presence that knows the stories that are arising in the mind's eye as fabrications while simultaneously opening one's *feeling awareness* to the effects that the energy of fear produces in the present-moment experience of the body. So we can see "Ah, there's the mind going off into the future again. Look at that," at the same time as inquiring, with a kind of conscious vulnerability, "How does fear *feel* right now?"

You will notice that the more space you can hold for the

energetic experience of fear in the present moment, the less power the thinking mind has to confuse and kidnap awareness. The center of attention shifts from the kaleidoscope of thoughts, perceptions, and images to the more palpable and immediate sensations of vibration, whirling, tightening, contracting (and, conversely, opening) on the level of the body itself. Bringing forth this kind of genuine interest in the present-moment sensations of fear isn't the end of the process, however. After all, who would want to just dwell in the feeling of fear for the rest of their life? The aim is to allow awareness to relate to fear in a way that frees us from its tyranny. You will notice that when you offer yourself this kind of sensitive attention and stay present with the *suchness* of fear—the actual feeling of it—another shift begins to occur: presence becomes free from its power. It becomes fearless in the face of it, knowing "This is fear. This is what it feels like. It's not bad or wrong. It doesn't mean it's going to be here forever. It feels this way right now. There's no need to make anything out of it." This fearlessness is not some kind of ego posturing, where you blast through things with a hard shell of apparent invulnerability. On the contrary, it is a humble kind of fearlessness that arises through the heartfelt willingness to be right here for your very natural human fear; to tremble with it and allow it to flow through the system, while trusting that your true home is always in awareness itself.

Through trusting in the power of awareness and allowing courage to guide your inquiry into the present moment, you are at the same time diminishing the power of fear itself. This doesn't mean getting rid of fear, but rather resting in a space of attention that is ready and willing to feel fear as fear without becoming a slave to the stories it tells or the contracted state it tries to lock you into. When fear is held in this way, with great kindness and a sense of how much you can hold and how much you can just leave be for now, you will notice that a gradual transformation takes place. Not having stories to feed on, the energy of fear becomes like the tentacle of a deep sea creature, looking for something to coil itself around. If you are patient with the flailing and thrashing and steadfast in the determination not to feed it more thought-food, you will also be present to delight in the refreshment that comes through the calming and ceasing of the energy itself.

Being present for the feeling of fear in this way is counterintuitive. As we have observed, there may be the sense that we need to keep it all hidden away so that it doesn't take us over. Of course, sometimes it can be helpful to focus on the bright, the positive, instead of fear itself, particularly if we are weak, lacking in capacity, or if we are taken over by the darkness that can accompany long-term illness. Balance is always important. You are your own guide in this process, and the most potent form of wisdom is your own intuitive sense of what the present moment needs. Trust that. However, exploring this direct way of allowing the energetic dimension of fear to be felt fully in the field of bodily presence is a powerful skill to cultivate. It begins to shift the ground of our presence itself. Out of this shift we discover a deeper capacity for transparency, kindness, and acceptance—all of which are essential allies when it comes to being with the difficulty, pain, and limitation that arise when we are ill.

ATTUNING TO DEEP TRUST

In addition to developing the capacity to be with fear as an energy occurring underneath the stories woven by our thinking minds, we can also explore its opposite: trust. As mentioned above, often we do need to turn our attention to a positive expression of heart, of being, in order to regain energy and vitality in our lives. However, as we looked at in relation to the quality of kindness, this doesn't refer to a manufactured state to try to push ourselves into or to cling to through willfulness—it is an inquiry directly into the heart-feeling of trust itself as an innate expression of our human being. Trust is a very useful antidote to states of fear that arise when the body isn't well, the mind is wiped out, or things aren't going the way you would like them to—in other words, when you realize the limits of your personal control over the conditions of life. The question is, what can you truly trust in?

Can you trust that conditions will always be the way you want them to be? Most of you who are reading this book already will have had a sobering insight into the reality that you can't. Even though consumer culture encourages you to orient your hope toward more comfort and convenience, more pleasant feelings, more material success, and dominion over conditions, you already know that this isn't a sure bet. Of course, for some of us, life can go this way for a time. In very rare cases, right up until old age—and then the cracks begin to show, sometimes shockingly and suddenly. For most of us it's a mixed bag—and for those of us who live with chronic illness, in that bag is a lot of stuff our ego definitely would not have chosen. You have already seen that physical health, pleasant conditions, and ego-oriented power can't ultimately be trusted in as a safe abiding place for awareness. No matter how much we cling, they change. Whether we want them to or not. So it is very useful to place our trust in that which is truly trustworthy—the simple perfection of presence itself.

Opening to this heart-feeling of trust in the inherent perfection of each moment, underneath all ideas, definitions, and self-images, is not the work of the analytical mind. Our analytical mind can only go so far when it comes to attuning to this dimension of experience. Reflective thought can point the way, but it is merely a springboard for the leap down and back into the heart itself. Opening to this kind of trust involves a faculty that is deeper yet simultaneously more direct, fresh, and vibrant than any concoction of ideas and concepts, and it arises through a sincere inquiry into the nature of awareness itself, as we will explore in more detail later in this book. In Buddhist traditions this quality of heart is often called Trust in Awakening, and refers to the deepest kind of trust we can have—the intuition that it is possible to wake up from the dream-state of continually generating the feeling that there is something wrong with this moment no matter how much apparent "evidence" our mind has gathered to support and solidify it. Not just in the future, but now. The Pali word *saddha* refers to this faculty of being and is often seen as the touchstone or foundation for other qualities that are praised in the Buddhist texts. It is important to note here that this kind of heart-trust needs to be balanced with wisdom and direct awareness so that it doesn't turn into blind faith or attempts to whitewash our experience with grandiose ideals. When this balance is present, we are more available to taste the subtle but liberating flavor of unconditional value and inherent OK-ness underneath the conditions that are manifesting in the present moment. If it remains a concept, it doesn't go very deep. You have to find it for yourself, in the heart of your own experience. There is no path that can be drawn to take you to this trust—all that can really be said is "Have a look for yourself."

What is it that doesn't come and go with the ups and downs of conditions? What is left when you let go of all ideas of who you are and what your illness means? What is it in you that can be aware, stable, and clear even in the midst of discomfort, fatigue, and disappointment? Even if you can only sense the seeds of this quality right now, the contemplation itself will be of great value and serve to diminish the hold that fear has on your mind. As we have seen, the arrow on the map doesn't point to the specific details of conditions, which are ever changing and often far from satisfying when it comes to even one day lived with the experience of illness. It points back to your here-and-now aware-ness itself. That is always the doorway to abiding in the safe harbor of trust in the timeless dimension right here underneath the conditions of body and mind. When we attune to this kind of trust, we simultaneously experience the blessing of other forms of inner strength—such as a confidence that we will be well-resourced enough to meet whatever arises in the future without being spun out into suffering. And we also know that if we are spun out, there is always a way back home to the safety of pure presence itself.

MEDITATION ON FEAR AND FEARLESSNESS

Relax into the position you are in now, or if you like, take some time to find a posture that will be comfortable for you. If your body is well enough, you may now be getting used to closing your eyes and sitting in a chair with your spine straight and your belly open, or even sitting on the floor in a meditation posture if you have the strength. If you are experiencing fatigue, weakness, and exhaustion, or the nature of your illness prohibits you from sitting upright, you may have found a position lying down in bed or on a couch that feels optimal for focusing your attention in-ward. All of these are perfect, keeping in mind that while pos-ture is a support for meditation, it is only that. The real work occurs in the field of your direct present-moment attention.

Take a few moments to bring your attention to the rhythm of the breath, still with your eyes open, reading the words on this page. Stop after this sentence and connect to the natural flow of breathing as you feel it in your body right now, no matter how subtle, coarse, deep, or shallow it is.

Have you found that capacity to be with the sensations of the breath, just as they are, without judgment, force, or losing focus? If so, just rest there for another few moments with your eyes closed, and open your eyes when it feels right. Put the book down if that feels good. Let as much time pass as you need.

Welcome back. Now, with your eyes open, still resting with the rhythm of breath as you feel it in the body, in this moment, notice what kinds of thoughts or preoccupations are taking you away from this moment, from really being with yourself and these words or from staying connected to your experience. It may help to look around the room, while still feeling for the overall flavor of your mind state or the thoughts that are demanding your attention. If in this investigation you discover that the quality of fear, worry, or anxiety is pulling your attention, then keep reading. If you feel quite at ease or if other kinds of thoughts and feelings are present, then continue with the meditation on your own, bringing to mind your own intimate reflections on the qualities of trust and awareness we have been exploring above.

If you find that there are thoughts, perceptions, or images that are concerned with or worried about the future, or if you are already feeling an undercurrent of fearful energy in your heart itself, keep reading. Pause and take your time with each sentence.

Still in a contemplative mode, ask the mind, with an inclination toward listening compassionately, "What are you afraid of?" Give yourself time to feel for and receive the answers that come up. Depending on what mood you are in, the mind may either bark an answer back immediately, such as "You know what I'm afraid of! I'm afraid of getting sicker!" or it may be numb, vague, and evasive. Either way, stay open and receptive, remembering that the content of mind can do whatever it likes. You are the presence that knows it. If the energy of fear is strong in the present moment, then you may not need to engage the storytelling mind at all—all that may be required is your gentle receptive presence and a willingness to hold the discomfort of fear in your body, just as it is. Be vulnerable to your own fear. It may be unpleasant, but there is nothing dangerous about it—it is just fear. How does it feel right now? Underneath the stories of what might happen, what you don't want to happen, or its flipside, the desperate grasping at what you really hope will happen, how does it feel to feel in this moment? Stand firm in your feeling presence. Be undefended in your sensitivity to fear and unwavering in your determination not to get caught in the details of the story.

In this deeper connection, attuning to the sensations of fear as a present-moment phenomenon that you can feel rippling, spiraling, pulling, or sinking, feel for that place in yourself that isn't doing any of that. Feel the fearless space that is already present as the knowingness itself. Can you sense that there is actually a vaster yet more direct dimension of your attention present right now? It isn't the energy of fear, but the space that witnesses it, the heart that can relate to it. What is it like to consciously rest attention on that space in yourself, as if you are making more room around the experience of fear? Close your eyes now and see if you can get a feeling for how that works, sensing that the space of your awareness is much vaster than fear but still resonating with the energy itself, free from any judgments or demands on your mind. Spend a few moments feeling for this possibility.

What did you notice? Was there a sense of release that naturally opened up in the center of your being when you discovered your capacity to be with fear but not be identified with it? Did you notice presence becoming unexpectedly energized through giving fear a safe space to just be itself in the body?

Now close your eyes again in this space, adding a softness and tenderness of heart to the mix. Hold the energy in your expanded space of awareness with a loving, kind attention, as if you are putting a compassionate arm around its shoulders and simply being there for it while it trembles and wobbles and shakes. Listen patiently, kindly, and with the strength of equanimity, but don't forget who you are. You are not defined by any story. "The future" is being fabricated by your mind right now. But you are always safe at home in the ground of awareness itself. Trust that.

ANGER AND FRUSTRATION

Before my body got really sick, the self-image I had was of a nice, peaceful guy. Quite cool with everything. Definitely spiritual. And not angry . . . no, no—that was *other people*. My perception of anger was that it was messy, stupid, and pointless, and you shouldn't feel it. You should just hold it all together and practice "letting go." Yet despite this tendency to repress and deny the actual reality of anger, illness made me realize what it actually is. As it turned out, it wasn't what I thought.

Of course, as with fear and other primal currents of energy in the human psyche that arise in the context of long-term illness or pain, believing in and acting out the stories anger spawns is very destructive to ourselves and others. Perhaps my repressive attitude toward anger itself was born of a fear of the power of anger when it is hooked into a story we believe to be real—such as "Life is unfair," "I hate my body," or "I hate myself." Indeed, as we have seen, the principle of the Middle Way holds true when it comes to navigating the terrain of anger and creating a space where the energy itself can be accepted, felt, and transmuted. When it comes to finding true well-being in the heart and mind, merely acting it out leaves us just as impotent as when we attempt to repress or deny it. Although we may relish the initial hit of power that floods the system, that power soon flips around and turns into fear, regret, or self-loathing. The mirroring principle of *karma* always holds true: whatever we intend to others, or life, that's what we will intend toward ourselves. Whatever we offer ourselves, that is what we will offer the world and the other beings with whom we share the planet.

WHAT IS ANGER?

Before we look into ways of handling the energy and stories of anger when they arise, it will be useful to get some perspective on what anger actually is. Rather than a force to be feared and denied or merely a default position for the reactive mind, it is possible to inquire into the essential principle of the energy and what it actually wants. On the level of causality, anger arises when things don't go our way—it is frustrated desire, turned on its head into the will to push away, destroy, or obliterate all obstacles to the objects of our wanting, be they states, feelings, acquisitions, or perceptions of ourselves in relation to others. In many ways illness itself is a great desire-frustrater. It creates frustration on the most basic level of bodily feeling: we want to feel good, but we don't. It creates frustration on the level of our social persona: we want to perform tasks in the way we always have or with the same degree of proficiency or energy that others do, but we can't. It creates frustration on the level of personal power: we want to be in control, but we're not. From the position of wisdom and the open heart, it is possible to meet the experience of physical pain and personal limitation with heartfelt acceptance, patience, and deepening insight into what is really true. This is where our journey into the experience of freedom is headed and is the wonderful promise of this inner work you are undertaking. Yet there is also the shadow side. Sometimes the ongoing experience of failure and unpleasantness can solidify into states of depression and resignation, while at other times they can spin the mind out into a frantic and desperate energy to control experience or fix ourselves. I would like to suggest that the basic energy of anger lies hidden underneath both of those shadow responses to the experience of illness. Resignation on one hand and desperation on the other are warped versions of acceptance and determination respectively. When they take us over, it is important to gather our awareness back into the present moment and take some time to feel what we actually feel rather than merely being caught in the apparent reality presented by our stories. When we pause and don't do anything about what we can't change—the facts of our experience in the present moment—we may begin to notice the simple fact that we don't like how we feel. This isn't evidence that we are a spiritual failure. It is the beginning of our journey into the heart of reality, just as it is.

Acknowledging that we don't like what we are feeling, in full awareness, is an act of honesty and a kind of liberation in itself. It frees us from the fantasy images of who we think we *should* be and how we should feel about things into the facts of the present moment. It liberates the mind from sugarcoating experience and trying to "cheer up" all the time, and instead opens up a pathway to reconnecting with a power much greater than the mind that tries to force ourselves into a happy spiritual state. Through this self-honesty we realize a deeper truth about the primal energy of anger: it is actually hidden power. Although this power initially gets directed through destructive channels or locked up in depressive stories, which only serve to increase the sense of separation and division in ourselves, we realize that underneath all of these distorted expressions is a simple desire for ground, for strength, for energy, and for inner power. That's all it ever is. When we learn the art of compassionately and patiently seeing through the apparent reality it presents—the "bad thing" out there in another person, a situation, our body, or ourselves—we can begin to taste the simple potency of the energy itself and allow it to become a force that strengthens and revitalizes rather than diminishes our core presence. We may be surprised to find that in the black sludge of hate and the burning fire of rage there lies true gold.

Through this process we discover that underneath the superficial expression of anger as the experience of not-wanting what is here, anger is also a deep kind of wanting: it wants strength. Can you sense the truth of that in yourself? Whenever you have been angry at someone or something, what is it that you wanted to reclaim? In my experience, it is usually some form of power, strength, autonomy, or freedom. So the essence of anger is a kind of longing for strength, yet for some reason the conditioned mind is wired to look for it in ways that ultimately don't lead to real strength of presence at all. That mind is wired to feed the energy into the channels of division and separation, which only make us feel worse in the long run. However, the initial impulse is just what it is—the raw, primal current of anger—and can actually contain very important seeds of wisdom and self-knowledge. In Indian and Tibetan traditions, the positive expressions of this energy are embodied in the archetypes of Kali and Mahakala respectively. These external representations of what is in fact a primal, universal spiritual energy are useful pointers to the strength of spirit that can be distilled from the transmuted energy of rage and anger.

Anger is not to be judged. It is there to be understood, felt, and liberated of its shadow of hatred, reactivity, and the intention to cause harm. Whenever we get a taste of this, there is a sense of returning back to wholeness. Rather than basing our practice of contemplation and awareness on an ideal of being "nice," we enter the gritty reality of the human psyche and allow it to show us our true strength. Through paying attention in this way we learn more about the boundaries we need, the actions we need to take, and the determination of spirit that life is calling us to manifest. Sometimes the destructive force of anger can be channeled positively into the power to stop doing something we know is causing ourselves harm, whether it be subtle or coarse, relational or internal. All of those are positive expressions of the energy of anger that can be of great service to our long-term well-being and freedom. Of course this work takes time, patience, and sensitivity. The energy of rage is very potent. Handling it can be disorienting and therefore requires a strong container of awareness and embodied presence. This is a lifetime's work, not a quick-fix technique. You alone need to trust your own intuitive sense of the right time to meet this energy as it is and the right time to focus more on states of well-being and relaxation. There will be times when you don't have a choice, though. The next section will provide you with tools for staying centered and present in the process.

MEETING ANGER DIRECTLY

Sometimes we just feel angry, and it's obvious. There is nothing we can do about it, and no technique or act of mental agility will make it go away. When this is the case, it is useful to generate more space and insight around the patterns of thought that are present—the mind spinning into tales about "What I did wrong," "What they shouldn't have done," or "When will this @#$*&% thing go away?!" When stories such as these rehash themselves endlessly in the mind's eye and contract the bodily system into states of fiery rage, the best thing you can do is come back to the body and create space to compassionately and patiently be with the burning.

Remember your capacity to be the embodied witness of all stories and all feelings. Every story that arises in the present moment is generated by your mind itself. Rather than being caught in the details, you can distill the essence, such as "Right now, I

feel angry." It is liberating to bring attention to the burning, pul-
sating, or churning sensations of anger as they arise in the field of
bodily presence in real time rather than being distracted by the
imperatives they generate or the sense of "the problem" somewhere out there in another person or the world or in here as
"me," "my body," and "my illness." It takes strength and a radical kind of courage, but you can do it. You may need to remove
yourself from a situation or create an environment of calm and
support on the external level first. That can help a great deal
when it comes to really seeing through the stories that anger is
generating and making space for the energy to move, burn, throb,
and finally settle into a space of presence itself. Other times all
you can do is witness the whole thing, story and all, while another part of you is fully caught in the whirlwind of rage—but
even that half-awareness will prevent you from being caught in
the dictates of the ego-mind and the ways it wants to act on anger
either externally or internally. You will have one eye on the true
refuge.

As the motility of my stomach got weaker and weaker, I
began to taste anger directly in the heart, mind, and body for the
first time in my life. Previously anger had been either buried
away, deep in consciousness, and spiritualized into denial or
self-righteousness (manifesting as Buddhist fundamentalism in
my first few zealous years as a monk), or had taken over my
mind in flashes of an almost altered state of consciousness where
I would blurt out an insult or say something cutting and cynical
without thinking about the consequences. I had never really felt
the phenomenon of anger in the directness of my own presence
or the intimacy of my own bodily experience before.

The Thai Forest tradition adheres to a very demanding dis-
cipline around the consumption of food. It is very challenging
and takes a lot of adjusting to, even for those with strong consti-
tutions. A nun or monk cannot choose what they eat but instead

are required to practice humbly and gratefully accepting what is offered and making do with not eating any food at all after midday. As an ideal, it seemed like such a beautiful thing to me. In my early twenties, while still at university, I recall seeing a photograph of a group of Western monks lined up in a row with their bowls tipped slightly, smiling gratefully at the little morsels being offered by grand-hearted folk. This beautiful photo affected me deeply. I thought, "Wow. What an amazingly peaceful life that must be. So serene, so carefree. Nothing to worry about." Indeed, there is a beautiful simplicity and reciprocal sharing of energy that comes through living in this way, and it has the power to open one up to a sacred dimension of humble thanksgiving, awe, and human connection on a very primary level of heart. It allows you to be open, soft, and vulnerable. A lot of my experience in the monastery did indeed turn out to reveal this wonderful possibility of being. The form itself distills the essence of human experience to its most basic facets: we need to care and be cared for. My materialist mind of fast-food scoffing and fridge raiding, unable to function in the peaceful setting of the monastery, gave way to a quiet appreciation for the simple blessings of life. Mostly.

There were other times when the practice of only accepting the food I was offered brought me to the limits of what I imagined was tolerable on the level of unpleasant feeling—both bodily and emotionally. Unfortunately, the range of foods that my physical system could tolerate had become very limited about five years into my experience of monastic life. Thankfully, eventually I was given an allowance for special food. This was a very rare exception and an example of the great kindness and pragmatism of my teachers, but there was a period just before that when the experience of lining up for the meal became akin to running a gauntlet. Some days there would be just enough food I was able to eat and be grateful for. And other days . . . well . . . there was some rice. Until I stopped being able to eat rice. It was on one series of those days, back to back, that I met rage *as rage* for the first time.

Loss of control is a big thing for the ego-mind. When it comes to the realm of bodily health, pleasant and unpleasant feeling, it really brings up the basic existential biases of our human condition. Many of you will have already met this deep edge of human experience in ways I can't imagine. For all of us, however, the general principle remains the same. We want to feel good. When we can't make that happen, it hits a nerve. The more total the loss of control, the deeper the reaction we feel. That's just the way it is. When you wake up feeling terrible or when your physical condition gets worse and you can't think straight; when you have to cancel your plans and give up your projects for a day, two days, or a week; when your twenties, supposedly the high point of your life, are spent exhausted in bed . . . the list could go on forever. So it is of great benefit to cultivate the capacity of presence to be there for what arises in our heart and meet it with clarity, wisdom, and great compassion for the universal nature of this human experience in all its flavors.

On those days, when I was already starving, I'd turn up to receive the meal for the day and realize with a heart-sinking feeling that most of what the good folk had offered us to eat would lead to a day sick on the floor. This loss of control ignited a primal rage so powerful in my being that all I could do was let it be there in my mind, body, and heart, all afternoon. For a few years, it was possible to see it as a challenge, remain equanimous, even enjoy the lightness of body that came through not eating. After the initial novelty wore off (and my body became depleted), it wasn't so much fun. It was hell. The most intense experience occurred during a period of retreat, when we would all go back to our huts alone to eat instead of gathering in the hall as normal. I vividly recall the walk up the hill in the hot Northern Californian sun, having realized that this day too would be a day without food. Initially there was a steely, masculine mind of determination, saying, "I can do this. Just be equanimous. Practice patience. Be grateful." As the slow uphill walk continued, the sheen of this spiritual willfulness began to fade. All of a sudden an intense flood of anger consumed my whole body. The primal urge to drop-kick my alms bowl into the forest took over. Images of hatred for the monastic form, the community—everything—consumed me like a nuclear explosion burning everything and everyone in my mind's eye and deep in my belly.

As I sat on a little chair inside my hut, something in me realized that there was no repressing that response. I didn't have the mental energy to apply any technique or method of positive thinking or even sit in meditation. The practice became "Sit here and burn." A torrent of rage flowed through body and mind. There was still just enough presence to know that the stories weren't real, however. To my surprise, this presence became more accessible the more I gave up trying to control the energy and instead allowed it to be itself. I felt a warrior-like spirit arising through me. It was violent, destructive, and impulsive, yes, but the more I allowed it to be, without doing anything about it, the more strength of presence there was. Although my mental energy was weak, there was another kind of energy, a more direct vitality, that felt fully alive.

In these situations, there is something in us that *knows* the Middle Way intuitively. It's not a technique or a nice philosophy—it's standing nakedly in the light of the real and remaining there. So rather than kicking down my door and screaming at the unsuspecting squirrels, I instead allowed that urge, that drive, that impulse, to be present without actually acting it out. As the afternoon wore on and the energy began to settle, I played with the energy itself using my imagination. I found that there can be a lot of power in allowing the energy not just to burn but actually flow through the whole system—including the mind and the personality. In a more compassionate space now, I asked it, "What do you want?" Instantly the energy body imagined picking up a chest of drawers and hurling it though the window, delighting in the power, the sound of breaking glass, the sheer annihilating force of the energy. The whole system felt better. In doing this I also found myself encountering an energy of denial that tried to hold back from experiencing the impulse of rage. For a moment the thought of "Oh no, you can't imagine that—that's *wrong*" arose, accompanied by a tightening and contracting around the chest and belly. And yet allowing the primal mind to complete itself in the safe space of imagination brought presence back to a state of equilibrium. Having met itself vulnerably, in an undefended self-honesty, the mind felt curiously satisfied.

I am not suggesting that everything became wonderful all of a sudden. I was still hungry and tired, and the thought of another day of no food seemed as awful as it had the day before. What did arise from that process of feeling the power of rage, however, was the power to make a decision, to act. In a way it was a call to be strong in my self-compassion and to get real about the actual needs of the body. As we have seen, strength and compassion are not opposites, but in reality rely upon each other. It is amazing to realize that the seeds of compassion and self-kindness can be found even within such primal expressions of the energy of anger. What followed was a series of meetings with my teachers Ajahn Pasanno and Ajahn Amaro, who suggested that maybe it would be better to actually get some food I could eat. In the mirror of their pragmatism, generosity, and compassion, I began a process of finding those same qualities for myself. Underneath the anger that occurred in my mind's eye was actually a more fundamental kind of love. A deep caring for bodily existence itself and a desire to manifest the strength needed to look after it. That strength was deeper than all the ideals of the "equanimous me" or the "good monk" that the ego-mind loved to fondle and tried to get off on. It was actually in tune with life itself rather than a self-image, an ideal, or a comparison with someone else's experience. Reality always has an intrinsic wisdom when we actually listen.

THE UNIVERSAL NATURE OF ANGER

This way of meeting anger directly in situations like the one above can apply to any reaction of ill will that you experience in the face of loss of control, frustration, or limitation on the level of physical wellness. It also applies to relational anger—the anger that can arise toward those people who are trying to help us get better, who are caring for us, feeling irritated by us, or are offering us untimely advice on "what we need to do" to get well, as we will see later in the book. Whatever the specific situation, however, it is helpful to get underneath the stories, which often flick between self-doubt and the feeling of *wrongness,* to externally directed dialogues or imagined arguments with others. Does this sound familiar? Rather than getting swept away in a torrent of once-removed fantasies about a future argument or what you should have said to someone in the recent past, it can help immensely to find and connect to the primary feeling in your direct embodied presence. You can ask yourself, "What *is* this?" and keep asking until you *feel* what it is. This is the work of awareness practice. Being interested in reality and true well-being of heart takes us deep into the nature of experience itself and allows us to discover its universal characteristics. Everyone has this stuff. It's part of being alive. When we attend to it in that way, a transformation begins to occur. The heart opens to the pain of anger and holds it with compassion. When we really feel anger as anger, we cannot help but notice how much it hurts.

From this direct noticing, compassion for the state of anger itself blossoms naturally, right in the heat of the fire. We feel the sting. We feel how anger chokes us and can make us insane. When this is directly sensed with the openness of nonjudgmental awareness, something in us wakes up. We remember that we are always here, right now. There is no problem. You could even say that the only problem is the sense of the problem. But even that isn't a problem.

Very often the stories around the experience of illness, pain, or limitation that are spinning out in our mind's eye can be boiled down to some form of anger. Whenever we realize "Ah, that's what this is. It's anger," there is a kind of opening up, relaxing, and harmonization that occurs, even if the feeling of anger is still present. There is a sense of reconnecting to a universal truth—a phenomenon that isn't actually a personal problem or a spiritual failing. When we reconnect to the fact that we are angry and that to feel anger is natural, we come back home to ourselves. It is part of the nature of this human mind, this human heart. In this process a quality of clarity and precision returns: we know what is here and what it is. A feeling of relaxation results by releasing the impulse to judge it or contract around the shame or guilt that believes our anger is so intensely personal, unique, or secret.

Relaxing this judgment also relaxes the tight clasp in the energy body that gives anger the power to narrow our entire subjective experience itself. When we are angry we feel as if the story we are caught in is the only important thing that ever was and ever will be. "Life would be great if it wasn't for *this thing*. I hate it. *Grrr.*" "This thing" becomes *the only thing*. It is an incredible magic trick that the mind performs, and it is not easy to snap out of. However, beginning with clarity, relaxing into nonjudgment, and feeling for the universal nature of the phenomenon of anger consecrates a space in awareness where our heart begins to open up again. Anger tends to transform in the face of self-honesty. The violence of anger wilts when it is seen as itself. Anger gets a bit sheepish—it doesn't like it when it's seen without its armor, its war paint, its battle cries, or its array of flashing weaponry. We see the naked person inside—vulnerable, unhappy, perhaps sad, often afraid.

What does it take to meet that person inside your own anger? It doesn't require judgment or trying to stop her or him from being angry. But meeting yourself without all that extra paraphernalia creates a space where real transformation and insight can take place—in your own way and in your own time.

You cannot know what you will discover when you meet your own experience of anger in this way. Each experience is unique. There may be times along your path when the intensity of the energy or the power of the stories requires the presence of another, such as a therapist or specialist in the field of trauma work. I wholeheartedly recommend that you honor the intuition to reach out if it arises. I myself have many times, both during my time as a monk and, in a deeper way, following my departure from the monastic lifestyle. I have never regretted listening to that pragmatic intuition. Sometimes we need to talk, to be heard, and to be in a safe relationship with another while these powerful forces are arising. Gradually you may get more of a sense of how you are wired and what your needs are, which is very useful in navigating the experience of long-term illness. You can begin to make fewer decisions that lead to your own suffering, physically and mentally, and learn to take care of yourself in a wholehearted way based on your own understanding and your unique situation. Being willing to listen as clearly and openly as you can without shaming the direct experience of anger away through ideals or comparisons with who you should be is the doorway to the arising of this honest, personal, and very real wisdom. You may find that meeting the personal as universal actually allows you to be more fully yourself.

MEDITATION ON MEETING ANGER
WITH COMPASSION

Allow yourself to find a position for the body that feels relaxed and comfortable and that lets you feel at home in yourself. Feel for a posture that brings about a sense of safety. It could be lying on your back on a bed in the ways we have looked at in the previous exercises or sitting comfortably in a chair. If the experience of anger or frustration is really strong, sometimes lying in a fetal position can bring about a feeling of being held in our own safe space of healing presence.

Take a few moments to relax. To breathe. To connect to the natural rhythm of the body breathing. Let yourself come back to that total simplicity. Just relax with the flow of that rhythm—allowing it to hold awareness with a sense of homecoming, a sense of safety and centeredness in the present moment.

Whatever is here, find that place in your heart that can be a good friend to it. This meditation is for those times when you know there is a sense of ill will, dislike, darkness, negativity, or anger present in some form. Being friendly toward all of that is a liberating act. Try it right now. Give yourself permission to be the observer, the curious witness to all the stories and images arising in your mind's eye in this moment. Notice the entire take that you have on life, on your illness. What is it like? What is it saying? Give yourself some time to enter this precious space of nonjudgment and friendliness together with the strength of steadfastness and presence you have been cultivating. Put down the book for a few moments now if you would like to go inside yourself in silence.

Now see if you can find the primary sense of "I don't like

this" underneath the stories in the mind and contraction in the body right now. Instead of blocking it, trying to think nice thoughts, or trying to stop it from happening, just let it be as it is. But *really* let it be as it is. Sense the current of feeling underneath all of the ideas and images in the mind's eye. Open up the space of awareness more and more to hold the whole of it. To feel the whole of it as a present-moment phenomenon in the entire bodily system. Feel it in the guts, in the heart. Can you feel your fists wanting to clench? Can you feel your jaw tensing? Can you feel any burning sensations—flushes of heat in your face perhaps?

Come back to the place of stability and refuge that always lies in the middle—in between following and repressing your thoughts. Be centered and strong in awareness, not identifying with the content of the stories anymore but instead opening that curious eye of direct sensitivity and witnessing to scan the whole body and hold the whole phenomenon of "I don't like this." Feel it in its totality. Let it burn. Let it move through you. Let it move and be itself. You can be right there with it. Nothing dies in the process. You are coming alive.

The stories might keep arising, but you can keep coming back to the present-moment sense of "I don't like this," "I hate this," or "This sucks." Feel that feeling. Where is the center of it? Go into the feeling itself. What does that feel like? It may be a sense of boiling and curdling or it could be a sense of "stuck." A sense of being held in and contracted and pushing against something. Trying to break something open. Feel the pain that's there in that, with compassion for yourself. Feel that core sense of *grrr* in a wider field of empathy for yourself in the present moment.

Allow your compassionate awareness to open to that. Let yourself be sensitive to the pain of it so that you are now recognizing the universal qualities of rage, anger, dislike, annoyance, irritation, and frustrated desire. Just stay there. Stay in the simplicity of it. The absolute, universal simplicity of this primal response in the human organism. Resonate with it. Inquire for yourself right now, "What is this? What does it want?" Let it open up and unfold. Let it speak to you. Get intimate with it. Go beyond words and listen with pure awareness. Try to keep coming back to the primary volition—the primary motivating force underneath all the details—again and again. What do you find there?

With a mind of inquiry and interest, a sense of innocence toward the phenomenon of anger, and a heart of compassion—feeling the pain right there—just sit with yourself in this new context. Keep coming out of the mind's spin. Rest at home in the reality of your experience right now. See what unfolds when you do that. You may even find a deep kind of love you have never known before.

6

Allowing Deep Rest

WHEN IT COMES TO living with the ongoing experience of illness or pain, giving ourselves time and space to rest deeply is
essential. It is well known how important sleep is for the rejuvenation of the cells of the body and our vital organs. Yet perhaps
it is not as well known how important consciously resting the
momentum of the seeking mind, the absorption in activity, and
the compulsive doing-ness that many of us get addicted to is
when it comes to healing and nourishing our core presence and
often the bodily system itself. This kind of nourishment of presence, of heart, of being-ness, is a vital part of finding an authentic sense of inner freedom in the midst of painful, depleted and
uncomfortable physical conditions.

Of course there are times when absorbing in activity or sensory objects is necessary and functional—both in terms of our
daily lives and as a pragmatic way of alleviating the discomfort
and unpleasantness that very often accompanies chronic physical illness. However, most of us have not been trained in the art
of deeply resting and may even have forgotten that it has any

value at all. Yet, as many of you will already know, the pain of being caught in the compulsive need to be doing, proving, and producing something becomes amplified when our energy is low, our physical capacity is limited, and our thinking mind is weak. We know we actually need to rest. Being caught in that twilight of disconnection where we feel like we should be doing something but we don't have the energy or the capacity is agonizing and emotionally draining. Instead of resting, we spin our wheels unnecessarily. It amplifies the existential suffering of the fact of being ill ("I wish this wasn't happening") and often activates the tendency to contract around feelings of wrongness or lack of worth ("I am a failure/I'm not who I used to be"). Through using the skills we have been learning, however, it is possible to deepen our proficiency at consciously unhooking from these assumptions and feeling the relief that comes when we allow ourselves to simply rest with ourselves as we are.

WHAT IS DEEP REST?

The kind of rest that is being described here may be unfamiliar to you, so it will be useful to clarify what I am pointing to before beginning to look at ways of bringing it about and using it to heal the mind and heart in the midst of the experience of illness. On the most fundamental level, you could say that it is the capacity to rest out of doing-ness and into being-ness itself. It is a process of unhooking from the compulsive drive toward activity and the underlying contraction of heart that propels attention into it. It is that deep relaxation and relief that comes when we can attune to the inherent OK-ness of the moment; when we allow that sense of being right here, at home in ourselves, to nourish and refresh our whole body and mind from the inside out. Resting deeply is one way of tasting the flavor of this nourishment of presence and ties into both the cultivation of authentic self-kindness and the practice of direct insight and inquiry that we will explore in more detail later in the book. This deep rest can take place in many ways that are suitable for our condition, where we are in our lives, and the strength and energy levels of the body. It can happen while the body is full of discomfort and the mind has no energy. It can happen while walking down the street and releasing the mind from its spinning and fabricating. It can be a conscious choice in the middle of a day of feeling quite good, coming from the intuition that resting out of the whirlwind of mind-made worlds would be truly healing. It can also be motivated by the pain and frustration that accompanies activity when we are ill for long periods of time. Whatever the situation, this capacity to rest deeply arises when we give ourselves permission to drop the concerns of daily life, the habitual momentum of becoming and striving, and offer ourselves a moment, a minute, or an hour of wholehearted downtime. This kind of rest is an offering of great kindness to ourselves, but it takes self-discipline and trust to create such space and time in our lives. If you are bedridden or in a wheelchair, there still may be something in you that resists just being here. It is natural for the mind to get caught in this resistance, and of course mental activity and creative pursuits can be of much pragmatic benefit when the bodily system is uncomfortable or depleted. However, to intuit the wisdom of resting deeply is transformative when it comes to finding presence and spiritual well-being in the midst of the experience of illness.

If the whole concept is disorienting or just unfamiliar to you, it may be useful to revisit the guided meditations in the first three chapters as an anchor for your awareness and to strengthen the faculties of presence, self-kindness, and equanimity in yourself. Those practices and skills are essential components in the art of resting deeply. In my own life, I found myself learning this way of being through circumstances of my body themselves—

exhaustion, cognitive weakness, and lack of sleep. It was like I was being asked to just rest. In the process I realized the great benefit that resting deeply can have in releasing the mind from the twilight of nagging feelings of failure, the tyranny of the inner critic, and comparisons with how the day "should be going." On account of being so exhausted, it became necessary to just lie down and unhook from all the outgoing channels of the mind and heart that I could only half prop up anyway. It relieved the feeling that "I should be able to, but I can't."

Do you recognize this from your own experience? Lying down and just being nobody, right here, with no direction, no need to force myself to be anyone or do anything, became an oasis in the middle of daily life. Sometimes it would just be for five minutes. Other times, when there was nothing I needed to get done, an hour spent resting deeply in this space could change the whole direction and outlook of the day. It still does. In many ways it is like meditation without the formal meditation part—a meditative awareness combined with a wholehearted surrender into the moment. Sometimes inquiry and insight can arise in this space, but at other times it is possible to just let everything be as it is and gently turn down the dials of doing-ness in the mind, body, and heart.

In contemplating this possibility, you may be getting in touch with a fear of being seen as lazy. As we have observed, our society doesn't value rest as much as it does production and output, and many of us have internalized this value system as a kind of fear of stopping, of not being productive, of hopping off the treadmill. There may be something in yourself that imagines it will mean failure, losing value, or "being lazy." However, allowing yourself space and time to deeply rest is not laziness—not in the way that we perceive it to be. The word has a pejorative connotation, which, for myself anyway, always brings up a feeling of "wrongness" in the mind and body. So what is this laziness we fear? As we have seen in the earlier example of acceptance not being equivalent to resignation, deep rest doesn't mean becoming impotent, limp, or losing our capacity for creativity. In fact, when we rest deeply, in full awareness, what we usually find is a flowering and rejuvenation of the energy of presence and the faculties of creativity and mental agility. However, there is a letting go that is required in the process. Because the gratification isn't instant, we can easily begin to doubt the process as it is just beginning to unfold. If we stick with it, the letting go that happens consciously, out of curiosity, and through really contacting what is here for us in the moment will take the mind back into a state of refreshment. In allowing deep rest, we don't lose our creativity or our ability to make things happen and get things done—we in fact revitalize the core of our being where the really good stuff comes from.

You may have noticed that if you do, do, do without ceasing, the quality of what you're doing gradually loses it sharpness, freshness, and shine. On the other hand, allowing yourself to rest deeply enables you to return to the simplicity of being from which you regain your vitality and true perspective. Rather than a resigned hopelessness, it is a process of gathering back into the power of a whole body and mind awareness free from the obsession with past and future or the need to qualify itself through activity. Paradoxically, activity that then arises is more in tune with our natural wisdom and talents. The benefits are far-reaching.

LEVELS OF REST

Attuning to this quality of deep rest in ourselves has three main components, which could be described as levels or even layers. They are three areas of our being that we can attend to with the intention to rest, to unhook, and to find ease in the present moment. As with all qualities of mind and heart, they interact and influence each other, so it is important not to conceive of them in too linear a fashion. However, for the purposes of description, they can be seen as three stages of rest that progress from our overall attitude, to contacting the direct experience of this moment, and then right into the heart-taste of presence itself behind the details and textures of conditions.

When considering the practice of allowing yourself to rest deeply, you will most likely come across a current of energy in the mind that is hooked into doing-ness. Before meeting the energy itself, it is useful to question the worldview or orientation of mind it is built upon. This is the first level of the practice of allowing yourself to rest deeply in an authentic way. As you have seen already, getting free from the apparent reality of the stories, attitudes, and perceptions in the thinking mind is an essential first step in a direct shift toward embodiment in the present moment. The stories that encircle awareness through perceptions of who you are, who you "should be," and how you are valued will often be the core of what perpetuates this momentum of compulsive doing-ness.

This first level of inquiry is directed toward two things, then: value and identity. In our society it is the norm to value ourselves for what we have done, what we can show others, and what external achievements we can point to. Of course this way of valuing ourselves can be very useful for our self-confidence, our feeling of contributing to the world, and using our talents and skills to be of service to others; however, it often becomes infected with the toxicity of a clinging that doesn't allow it to rest. If our entire way of valuing ourselves is oriented toward achievement, production, and what we can *do*, then the experience of being ill, incapacitated, or depleted becomes agonizing. The flipside of only valuing ourselves through an image of being successful, useful, or achieving something is that we feel useless, worthless, and hollow when we are just here, being ourselves. While seeking value through an image tied into the doing-ness that can manifest in a day, a week, or a year has its place, it is also limiting and confining when it comes to experiencing a real sense of freedom in the heart. Undoing this habit and questioning the assumptions it is built upon is the work of spiritual inquiry and brings us right into the fabric of the present moment in an empowering and heart-opening way.

In the early Buddhist teachings, there is a wonderful word that encapsulates this dimension of ourselves when it is infected with clinging. In the Buddha's very first teaching, he described a mechanism in the mind, "the thirst to become," or *bhava tanha* in Pali, as one of the causes of the unnecessary suffering we generate in our human hearts and minds. Exploring this matrix of becoming and having the courage to unpack, unfold, and release its grip on our awareness gives us a powerful way of resting deeply in the moment. Can you recognize this force, this trance that your mind gets kidnapped by? It is that which fabricates images of yourself in other people's eyes and imagines them assessing you on how you are performing. It is inside the images of yourself that get wedded to systems of valuing that you have either internalized from society or constructed yourself throughout your life as a parent, an employee, a spouse, and so on. It is that habit of departing from the open, undefined nature of awareness and into a trance of unworthiness, lack, or images of yourself as deficient, followed by seeking to *become* a person who isn't those things by proving yourself through your activity. When the mind is caught in this matrix of becoming, resting deeply seems like another wasted opportunity that could be used to become the person we *should* be. What we don't see is that the seeking, thirsting, and hankering for value through a fixed image of ourselves is the present-moment cause of the loss of connection to a more sustainable kind of value. It is a contraction and an illusion that takes us out of ourselves, while subconsciously promising us that it is heading toward some kind of real ground. Within this trance, we forget the potential to feel valuable through simply being. We lose the taste of unconditional, inherent value that is available when we stop, unhook, and rest deeply into the heart itself.

Seeing through and unhooking from the stories of becoming in the mind's eye is a choice, not an obligation. Nor is it an absolute stance about doing-ness, creativity, and using our skills to benefit the world. As with all of the practices in this book, its potency lies in how appropriate it is to the present-moment condition of your mind and its efficacy in clearing a path for inner well-being and freedom of heart. Not even these frameworks can be clung to. They are merely pointers. I say this here, as it is important not to generate an internal aversion or judgment toward activity itself, which is just a shadowy way of still being caught in its vortex and doesn't liberate the heart to rest deeply. As you have probably sensed in your own life already, the stories of becoming can be both intoxicating and crushing. Freeing the mind from clinging to and seeking our identity through the intoxication doesn't mean hating it. If we look honestly in the present moment, we see that in fact taking a position against activity is another kind of becoming itself, what the Buddha astutely called "the thirst to not-be," or *vibhava tanha* in Pali. The stories of becoming can be destructive and focused on repression as well as seeking satisfaction through propping up a self-image. Being ill can generate negative stories of becoming in many ways, and a subtle shadow side of spiritual inquiry can be a negativity directed toward the everyday, functional becoming that sustains us and is in fact a necessary part of being a human being. We can't become a nobody. So, in inquiring into the influence that *becoming* has in inhibiting your capacity to rest deeply in the present moment, I would encourage you to remain open and free from judgment. Make it a personal inquiry. Get curious.

The second layer of rest occurs in the energetic field of the body as it is sensed in the present moment. The process of allowing ourselves to rest deeply involves a conscious relaxation and letting go on the level of our bodily presence itself. It is a process of easing and releasing the gripping, holding, and tightening than can become second nature to the way we relate to our bodies. It can be useful to use the body-scan technique we have already explored, deep breathing, or somatic practices such as restorative yoga to enhance the sense of connection to our body, just as it is, in the present moment. On this level, we are looking to feel for a direct sense of relaxation in our limbs, our belly, our face, our legs, and, most important, the mental posture in which we are holding the body in awareness. In inclining toward an attitude of relaxation and openness, we may encounter a kind of restlessness or agitation that is hooked in to certain objects of activity—the internet, the day's projects, communications with others, or just the unquestioned assumption that we need to be constantly doing something to feel alive. There can be a residual buildup of this restless energy that may have been accumulating for a lifetime, so it is important to find ways of gently unfolding it and feeling for other possibilities of relating to the present-moment experience of being in your uniquely wired human body. On the energetic level, this kind of experience is the result of patterns of attention that we may have been reinforcing for a very long time, so it is important to create a space of patience and nonjudgment around their very arising. It is possible to relax alongside these forces themselves. As with all these practices, the quality of awareness you bring to the moment will determine the long-term results. Sometimes all we can do is relax around that which is agitated. This tends to have a calming effect on the system, and the anxious, frantic energies in the system have a space in which to unfold in their own time. The possibility of allowing yourself to relax in this way lies in the sensitivity and responsiveness you bring to the experience. It forms the basis of a feeling of trust that being here, just as you are, is nothing to fear. Connecting to this trust will allow you to experiment with putting things down and consciously relaxing the hold that your mind has on the body and the hold that the state of your body has on your mind.

However, it is also important to acknowledge that sometimes being here with the body in the midst of illness or pain is the hardest thing in the world. There are levels of discomfort and unpleasantness that can arise that are way above and beyond our current threshold of awareness. It is up to us to know these for ourselves. We all have an internal gauge of what we can and cannot be with, let alone rest deeply into, and it is important to start from where we are. If the levels of pain, discomfort, or the overall feeling of "yuck" are pushing the meter into the red zone, then resting with the experience of the body in this direct way sometimes can heighten the sensations and become overwhelming. I would recommend dipping a toe into the process, though, as there are other times when we can be surprised by a sudden dropping away of the intensity of discomfort itself. It is like the clouds suddenly part when the attention and intention of the mind unwinds and lets go. As you exercise this faculty more and more, you will find that the capacity to rest with experience as it is increases. But you alone know the right and the wrong time for this, so please listen to what your intuition tells you. Don't try to force yourself to rest. You will only get more force and less rest. There is no succeeding or failing here. If you can't rest with the body right now, honor that. You are not wrong.

The third layer of this process of rest is a key piece of what differentiates it from the usual kind of rest that turns it into sleep. While the excellence of a short, deep power nap is nothing to be scoffed at, what we are looking to cultivate here is the capacity to rest deeply while we are fully aware. This full awareness isn't a cognitive busyness or even a heightened state, but rather what arises when we engage in the process with an interest and a spaciousness that can witness phenomena in the present moment with openhearted objectivity. As we have already explored, this dimension of ourselves is always here and now, yet is also the easiest thing to overlook. Resting deeply in this way involves an orientation that is simultaneously attentive to the content of experience and curious about the ground of presence itself. This curiosity is what allows us to unhook from compulsive becoming energy and to soften the edges of restlessness or walled-off-ness through the present-moment input of wholehearted caring and self-kindness. Without it, our time of rest will quickly be co-opted by waves of alpha state imagery, a soporific flood of chemicals, and finally deep sleep. While that latter process is of course of benefit when we need to sleep, it doesn't lead to a new way of being, and we don't get to meet our mind and heart directly. We just zone out. Resting deeply into the feeling experience of presence and finding our home there is of a different nature. It is a gradual unfolding of the momentum of doing-ness into a place in ourselves that feels unconditionally OK. Through consciously unbinding awareness from its self-measurements, comparisons, and the search for value through becoming something or someone, we taste that quiet but profound value that lies within simply being.

BEING PERFECTLY EXHAUSTED

Of course, sometimes when you realize you need to rest deeply, it is because you are actually exhausted. When the body is weak and our resources are limited, all the pushing, making, changing, and planning that can consume our daily lives can wipe us out very quickly. However, when we actually come to rest, there is often a subtle judging that is present—a feeling of failure, or a sense that "I'm exhausted again. It's my fault. What have I done to cause this?"—and attention can then become preoccupied with trying to figure things out through the thinking mind. So even while we are entering consciously into the process of rest, something in us can be impeding the process by dividing itself off from what is actually happening. When I notice this in myself, I like to explore what it feels like to totally get with what is here. Sometimes using the verbal faculty in my mind's eye can be a useful way of initiating a shift of being in this way. For example, one phrase that I have found useful is "I'm doing exhaustion perfectly right now. I'm perfectly exhausted." Although these are just words, they can actually help to bring a smile to the heart and to precipitate the feeling sense of relaxing into the suchness of the moment without self-blame or subtly dividing ourselves from it. Of course I'm not really "doing" exhaustion—it is just the condition of the mind and body—but this kind of reframing of the very perception of what is happening can help bring balance and the sense of rightness back into the moment. It is perfectly what it is. In recognizing this, our being feels whole again. By using such words and phrases (which are always most potent if they arise spontaneously in relation to the present-moment experience), the heart remembers the possibility of being one with the experience of the body rather than split off in an abstract realm of commentary, criticism, or resistance. Often this unity with the exhaustion that is present can bring about a deep shift in the felt sense of the body, as we bring our attention to it in a soft, open, but clear way.

Try it now and see how it feels. If exhaustion and fatigue are here right now, feel what it is like to embody them perfectly. Use whatever words or phrases come to mind to help relax out of the inner critic or the conviction that things are going wrong. Instead, say "yes" to the experience of tiredness and use the softening that comes about to relax into a rested feeling of presence.

UNFOLDING THE STORIES OF BECOMING

While at times the inner obstacles to resting deeply can be based primarily on the feeling tone of the body, as we will explore soon, there are often psychological obstructions that we might not have the tools to recognize. These are often wedded to the stories and energetic currents enmeshed in *becoming,* as we have looked at briefly earlier. The basic template for understanding both this energy in the mind and the stories it spawns lies in the word itself. From the perspective of our true nature, the inherent wholeness of presence, right here and now, any kind of becoming is a movement away from what we already are in this moment. The mind gets conditioned to seek identity and satisfaction through channels of becoming from very early on in our lives. While in itself this is a benign and often useful creative force, when it is not seen for what it is it can enslave us and keep us trapped in very limited assumptions of identity or rules of what is acceptable and what is not. One form of this inner entrapment is the feeling that we need to measure our value through becoming somebody or something other than what we are right now. Somebody special maybe. Or perhaps somebody who has it all under control, who is winning, or who isn't weak. Of course, we are always ourselves, but in our mind's eye we can find ourselves habitually comparing an image of ourselves to an image of someone else and trying to extract a feeling of value from that. Or we may have the kind of mind that continuously doubts the images we have of ourselves and hops from one image to another—still in search of the elusive feeling of value, of ground,

FINDING FREEDOM IN ILLNESS

and ultimately of having a resting place for the heart. However, you may have noticed in your own experience that this never happens. As the very images our attention is trying to rest upon and identify with are themselves mind-made, they are also sub-ject to change, to cease, to morph, and to warp. There is no rest-ing place in the whirlwind of endless becoming, no matter how hard we try to make it so. When it comes to the possibility of allowing ourselves to rest, this force in the mind can generate stories of doubt, fear, or holding back that prevent us from really surrendering deeply into the process. It is useful, therefore, to become wise to the kinds of stories that take over the mind when we incline toward rest deeply, here and now.

I recall one time in my life when I really had to meet the energy and the stories of this *becoming* energy in full force. It was after I had decided to leave the life of a monk, knowing in-tuitively that a change of lifestyle was needed in order to offer my body the compassion and care that it needed for healing to take place. There was a period of about a year following my departure from the form of monastic life and the very clearly defined roles therein when I was just no one. I had no job and had very little experience of adult life outside of the monastic setting. There was nothing I felt inspired to do, and I knew what was really needed was to wait—to just rest in the unknown and allow life to move through me. However, another part of me didn't like this at all. While my intuitive sense of wisdom knew that I needed at least a year to just rest, deeply and fully, the momentum of becoming that had been hiding within the iden-tity of "monk" began to flail around in consciousness, thirsty for a new self-image to hold on to. It didn't like the vast uncer-tainty ahead. It wanted to *be someone . . . now*! After a few days of being tormented by endless stories of "What I could do, and who I could be, and what if I did such-and-such, and maybe I'll go to university again, . . ." I decided that the kindest thing I

118

could do for myself was to make space around the stories that were galloping through my thinking mind and whirring through the energy body. While the stories were compelling and seemed to offer some form of solace from the discomfort of not knowing who I was anymore, I could sense a flipside that was perhaps more painful: the very real possibility of losing connection to the peace of presence and charging forward into projects and schemes that I sensed would hinder the healing process that had begun. Thankfully, the longing to get better and really take the time to rest was stronger than the strategies the mind was conjuring up to allay feelings of insecurity, lack of value, and being useless. A space opened up that allowed awareness to be with those stories and really listen to what they were saying rather than blindly following them and ending up severed from the healing process I had very tentatively entered into.

I noticed that the subtext of all the stories that presented themselves, all the plans and schemes about "Who I could become," was an assumption that just being here, breathing, aware of the body was not enough. There was a feeling that "I need to become somebody . . . or . . . or . . . I have no value." In hindsight, the necessity to stop and rest was at this time a great gift— I felt my attention getting alongside these stories in the mind, including their opposite, such as, "You're a loser. You've failed," and allowing the heart to really feel the pain of being locked into that mind-set.

At times the force of the energy that arose was so strong I literally felt myself holding onto my chair, as if to prevent myself from lunging out into some kind of project based on fear. Indeed, at the core of the stories that arose was very often fear, pure and simple. Coming back to that direct energetic sense in the body itself, as we have already seen, is a powerful way of coming out of the spin of the mind's resistance to deep rest. "Ah, this is fear," I came to know gradually. Through gently but consistently being with the feeling of fear, I began to ask my mind, my heart, some questions. "What are you really afraid of?" I found myself asking in my mind's eye. "I'm afraid that if I just rest here and do nothing it will mean I am no good" came the reply. "No good?" I asked. "Yeah . . ."

In the process I began to meet something very old in the heart, in my psyche itself—an old conditioned assumption that who I am right now, without any appendage attached, any mask of becoming to refer to, is probably not quite right. It's probably wrong in some way. The voice that spoke was childlike and shy, but it was a beautiful meeting that took place. Days were spent holding that tender feeling in a space of compassion and inwardly directed warmth. Other days required a more masculine quality of saying "Nope. Not gonna follow you" to the stories of becoming and the agitated, fragmented energy they generated. Gradually the compulsive resistance to the space of deep rest I had created began to loosen its grip, allowing the heart and mind to rest with the body just as it was. A kind of harmonization began to emerge as I allowed myself to surrender to the process rather than second-guess it, fight it, or restlessly twiddle my thumbs waiting for it to be over. Compassionately and clearly releasing from the stories of compulsive *becoming* in the mind was crucial to that process. It allowed both a healing of the body and an opening of the mind to take place.

After several months had passed, I began to feel a state of equilibrium and a trust that it was the right time for activity. This trust came from a shift that had arisen in my motivation. No longer was it a desperate need to escape the uncertainty and unknown quality that accompanied this time of healing—it was rather an interest in offering, in creating, and in sharing that was coming from my center rather than kidnapping awareness and forcing me into becoming something. The difference between the two is obvious when we look into the mind and heart.

While compulsive *becoming* is motivated by fear and a conviction about our own lack of value, the creativity that emerges from a space of presence and wholeness comes from love, enjoyment, and a spirit of offering and sharing. It was only through allowing myself the time to rest deeply and give the body space to begin a process of healing that the possibility of this new kind of doing-ness arose. While for all of us it can and does get co-opted by the shadow side of clinging, the comparing mind, and the need to become someone in the eyes of others, we can always find our way back to what is true if we give ourselves the time to rest deeply out of the mind's addiction to becoming.

RELAXING IS CARING

The quality of relaxation that is involved in conscious rest can begin to bring forth another kind of energy: one that is rich, settled, and connected to an inner sense of deep caring for yourself. This energy of caring is the positive heart-resonance that flows forth from the intention to rest. In a way, conscious resting *is* caring. When we do this we connect to a hidden resource of compassion and wisdom in ourselves—one that bestows a simple loving presence onto the entire field of experience because it feels the value and *rightness* of that. It is an expression of taking care of ourselves intimately. This positive dimension of being that can emerge has similar qualities to the energy that mothers have for their children—that warm, open, unconditional offering of presence. That same kind of fullness of heart flows forth when we allow our attention to loosen its grip, to soften its holding, and to relax into the sensations of this very moment. It is a universal potential in us and one that we really need when the body is unwell, vulnerable, and broken. The magic is that we can offer it to ourselves in a wholehearted way that actually brings about a shift of the energetic state in the present moment.

It isn't just a nice idea or a theory—it is the core feeling of loving and caring for this bodily form, in whatever state it is, that quite naturally accompanies the intention to soak deeply in conscious rest. When we approach it this way, we begin to experience a subtle feeling of enjoyment. It isn't the same kind of enjoyment that comes from being outwardly oriented on the level of the senses, but is something quieter, something more deliciously intimate and healing to the fabric of body and mind. The energy of caring and relaxing through self-kindness and trust can give rise to a gentle suffusion of inner pleasure, even when our body is weak and in pain or our thinking mind is muddy, exhausted, and confused. This is the pleasure of presence itself when it is freed from tightness, holding, and hardening around the here-and-now experience of the body.

UNDOING INNER DOING

Although we have looked at ways of shining a light on that habit of mind that believes it can only have value through external activity and the forms of becoming that accompany it, there is another kind of internal doing-ness that is also very useful to relax in this process of deep rest. It is the compulsion to fix, change, or modify the experience of this moment in some way—to get somewhere or be something in our mind's eye itself. When it comes to conscious rest, this internal level of activity can also be relaxed, through using presence itself as our frame of reference. The more we explore this presence, the more we discover the unconditional fact of its existence. It is here, despite what is going on in the body or the mind. In dark states, it is here. In states of joy and bliss, it is still here. It can't be grasped conceptually—and that isn't the point anyway. The point is to learn the art of finding true ground in the subtle aliveness and peace of that presence itself. One of the ways of bringing this about is through deliberately relaxing the mind that is looking to make something out of this moment. The one that is trying to make it better, or higher, or deeper.

This force in the mind is the same drive of becoming we have already looked at in its most primary form. Once we have relaxed the compulsion to be doing something externally, through the body and the senses, the internal momentum of this becoming energy itself often takes new objects based on the process of meditative rest itself. When we get quiet, extend presence throughout the body, and commit to just being here, we will meet a deeper layer of doing-ness in the mind and heart. If it remains unseen, then the process of rest can get kidnapped by all sorts of complications, self-measurements, and, sadly, more stress. We may notice thoughts and images such as "I'm not resting as well as I should be," followed by "I bet other people do this better than me," and then "If it weren't for this [insert particular feeling or symptom of the body here], I would actually be able to rest." These fabricated assessments of the present-moment process can seem very compelling and real, but in fact they are just more subtle ways of avoiding the simplicity of resting here with this moment. In our spacious but determined awareness they can be gently undone, unfolded, and relaxed. They are not necessary. Presence is always already here. The stories that this kind of internal doing-ness generate can present themselves as potential remedies for the absence of rest, such as "If I just fix this, change this, think about this some more, then I'll be able to rest," yet in reality they are actually the cause of internal agitation themselves. They are ways of not resting here with the moment. They are departures from the here-and-now presence that can really heal.

In your own explorations and experiments with allowing yourself to rest deeply, you may come across many different varieties of this kind of internal struggle to do, to make, or to fix.

Whatever the content of the stories, the art is to trust in doing as little as possible, in full awareness, in this moment. You don't need to make the process complicated. You can un-complicate it. This unfolding and unbinding can go deeper and deeper as the energy of presence becomes more palpable in your body and mind. It is like riding a bike. When the bike gets going, you don't need training wheels anymore. You are riding. While initially there will be forms of doing-ness that aid the process—such as establishing intention, resting with the breath, or gently going through a body scan meditation—eventually the feeling of presence pervades and suffuses the present moment and provides a contrast to the stray impulses of inner activity that pull us away from it.

MEDITATION ON DEEP REST

For this meditation, I recommend that you use the lying down posture we discussed on pages 25–26. However, if you have physical limitations that prevent this, please find a posture that is in harmony with your condition and opens you into a similar feeling of letting go and rest.

Take a few moments to settle into the lying down or resting posture you have chosen. Allow yourself to fully appreciate the sense of relief that comes through lifting the pressure off the body. In this meditation on rest we are consciously relaxing that sense of pressure, beginning with the body itself. Let yourself relax the burden of needing to hold the body together, keep it upright, or move around.

Give yourself permission to enjoy the pleasant feeling of lying down just for its own sake. Enjoy the shift of bodily sensations that it brings about.

This may mean feeling for the *relative* pleasure. If you have a lot of pain, for example, then you can still focus on the relative easing of discomfort that comes about through relaxing the physical posture in this way. Feel that shift in yourself, no matter how humble.

You may need to experiment with adjusting the posture to get a sense of this. See if you can find that "sweet spot"—that one posture that feels like, "*Ahh*, I can relax now." Give yourself time to find it. Drop the ideas of what meditation *should* look like—and feel for what posture activates that sense of coming home, of rest, of ease for you. Be creative and free with this bodily inquiry. This exercise has a very primal quality to it. It's almost like coming back into the womb—a place where we feel protected, safe, and held within a sphere of protection. See if you can wholeheartedly and generously offer yourself that as you lie here.

Relax any sense of holding back or embarrassment even—allow yourself to be vulnerable to yourself. And allow that vulnerability to inform your decisions on how and where to let go and how to be with your unique body right now.

Now close your eyes and give yourself a few moments to feel how this feeds back into your mind state itself. Can you feel a relaxation that seeps into your energy system, your inner sense of yourself? Give yourself some time to fully enjoy that feeling. Drink it in.

You can put the book down now and take as much time as you like to explore this process for yourself before opening your eyes again.

Now bring forth a quality of friendliness and a gentle attitude of caring to your whole physical being. With your spacious awareness, gently encompass the places that feel painful, stuck, tense, dead, numb, or even shut down. See if you can allow your awareness to meet these too as you rest with the breath and the pleasant sense of gravity holding the body in its arms. Soften and relax around what you may usually try to get rid of, those unwanted experiences. Can these too be welcomed into this field of conscious rest? There is no need to push away, pull back, or contract around the discomfort that is present. Feel what it is like to meet it with no interpretation at all—no measurement, no conclusion—it is just this. How does that shift of attitude affect your mind state?

With this sense of friendliness and kindness you can be present alongside the afflicted or the broken. There's no need to force yourself to make it change, to fix it, or get rid of it. Instead attune to an all-around feeling of relaxation. Attend to how you can stay with it and not push past where the body needs to be right now. Stay with a broad spacious awareness. Attend to rest itself.

Close your eyes now as you deepen the process of letting go, and take your time to feel the sensations that come with it.

Attuning to a deeper level now, see if you can sense in the present moment the desire to become someone or something. Consciously relax the outgoing tendencies—thinking about things you have to do or subtle voices telling you that you are being indulgent or lazy. Put down all the tasks and agendas of everyday life. Consecrate this time for deep rest, intimately and fully. Give those tendencies space—but don't buy into them. They are just the murmurings of the conditioned mind.

Let the concerns, the worries, and the stories around the future just rest. Unplug yourself from the spin of compulsive doing-ness or needing to be something or someone and focus on drinking in the refreshment of wholehearted deep rest. Feel the healing that is activated when you do that.

As you attune to this quality of deep rest, you can also sense what it brings about in the heart or the mind—a quality of refreshment and release perhaps—without needing to do anything at all. This is the beauty of this simple meditation. The quality of deep rest *is* your object. Allow it to suffuse the whole body.

Let it permeate your intentions and the heart of the mind itself. Let this new orientation transform the energy that the mind itself arises out of.

Feel if you can unbind the mind and heart from obsession with doing-ness around the meditation itself in this moment. What if this moment is just this moment? What if the need to understand it, define it, and make it a "success" is relaxed? How does it feel to undo this level of doing-ness in the heart and mind? What does it take to trust that you are completely allowed to rest here as presence itself regardless of what the body is feeling or the thinking mind is doing?

Drink in that beautiful feeling of deep rest. Allow the dials in the mind to move slowly toward zero. Rest as presence itself.

Close your eyes now, and take as long as you like for the process of deep rest to do its healing work.

7

The Heart of Relationship

WE LIVE IN the age of the individual. Urbanization and tech-
nology have enabled us to imagine, more than ever before, that
we live our lives in a hermetically sealed container of "me." No
longer do we meet the people who grow our food—we pick it
out from long aisles in sprawling, brightly lit warehouses. No
longer do we learn about our world through conversations, but
through sound bites and pixels emanating from our myriad de-
vices. We are encouraged to compete, to make it for ourselves, to
get ahead of the others, and to win. While social media is in
many ways rekindling the art of conversation and interdependence, it often feeds this culture of individualism as well. We are
encouraged to have "followers" and "fans," and in many ways
the once-removed wall of the computer screen can bolster our
narcissistic tendencies rather than create a real feeling of connection, vulnerability, and openness. This apparent ability to
seal ourselves off from the world comes crashing down when we
get sick. We realize that we can't do this on our own. We need
others to hold us up—physically, emotionally, and perhaps even

financially. For many of us this can feel like a rude awakening. Perhaps for the first time in our lives we are faced with the prospect of becoming dependent on another person, on our family, or our community. This can be an immensely trying and humbling process if we have spent most of our lives unconsciously feeding the illusion of being "above it all." Sadly, if illness comes very late in life, some of us can resist the process of opening to the love, care, and support of others until the very end. When we do this we also miss out on the profound beauty that comes forth when we begin to open to the field of interrelatedness and connection that has in fact always been a part of our lives.

MEETING THE WALL

For most of us who go through periods of chronic or long-term illness, there comes a time when we meet a wall in ourselves. This wall is that within us which resists allowing others to see our vulnerability, to pick us up when we are down, or to help us do what we can't. It is a relational wall—one that we have perhaps built up over a lifetime, for many practical reasons. When we are living a life of physical health and energy, it is important and pleasant to feel the relative freedom that comes with independence, personal power, and the ability to make things happen through our own effort and creative energy. It's fun, it generates self-respect, and allows us to do well in our lives. Yet this capacity can easily create biases and tendencies in our hearts that serve to prop up an illusion of invulnerability, complete autonomy, and separation from others. When our physical health and energy are depleted or compromised, we experience the shadow side of these biases as a wall in the heart. Our presence hits up against it, and it hurts. For some of us it can become apparent through feelings of embarrassment or shame that arise when there is no choice but to let others help us get out of bed, do our laundry or other such everyday tasks we may have taken for granted. Even little things such as accepting a cup of tea from a loved one when we're crashed out on a couch or in bed may bring these feelings up, sometimes overwhelmingly. Although I have never had to be showered or dressed or have a catheter changed, I have heard many tales of the challenge of this type of experience—of suddenly being dropped into a realm of naked vulnerability—from those I have worked with. For some of us the wall may come up as feelings of resentment and irritation toward others as they extend their generosity toward us. If our particular bias is pride, it can feel like an affront to our ego to have to accept the help of another in such basic and potentially intimate ways. When this tendency is left unchecked, it can lead to stubbornness and tyrannizing ourselves with unrealistic expectations of what we "should" be able to do. If the reality is that we actually *can't,* and we know it, deep down, the results can be very unfortunate—both on the obvious physical level and the internal level of self-care and mental well-being. Refusing and resenting the help of others through subtle feelings of bitterness or unquestioned anger at the universe, or God, or life, only makes the heart more contracted and in the long run will actually increase the overall sense of the suffering of our predicament.

As we have seen, the contracted heart is a guarantee for the amplification of pain, the feeling of stuck-ness, and mental suffering. Although it may seem like it is protecting us, it is actually blocking out the light that shines in as the walls begin to dissolve. Letting in the sunlight of our simple human connectedness is a miracle in itself. It is a kind of beauty that we can experience even in the midst of losing personal control or during moments of great vulnerability and dependence upon others.

One of the first walls in my own heart that came to light when my capacity for autonomy and personal power on the physical level began to dwindle was the idea that allowing myself to depend upon others meant becoming weak. Having been so used to living with the relative strength that came from willpower and the assumption that the less I needed from anyone, the better I was doing, this was understandable. Even in the context of the interdependence that is part of the monastic form, I managed to keep feeding this sense of separation, perhaps even amplifying it in many ways. My ego could get off on the sense that I didn't need anything from the world, I didn't even need money—I was *really* independent now. Of course, this assumption was farcical, as my entire existence in that peaceful setting depended upon the daily generosity of the kind folks who brought us food and paid to keep the whole place running. It is humbling to realize now how the mind can resist what is so obvious, even in a setting deliberately designed to bring about an appreciation of the blessings of interconnectedness and mutual support. Born from this skewed obsession with personal independence was an underlying fear that letting others in meant losing power and safety. This is a normal disposition for many of us, isn't it? We feel that if we let down our guard and open up to the feeling of being held, we will get hurt or be taken advantage of. Of course there are times and places where this kind of vulnerability is not what is called for, as we will see, and in some cases it indeed may not be the wisest mode of being. We always have a choice. However, when we forget this ability to choose, we feel that we have no option, and there is no way for the wall to come down. We don't know how to let it become porous or even dissolve. This is a painful state of being.

This habit of equating interpersonal vulnerability with weakness can bring about many other kinds of suffering in the heart. As my own ability to prop up the illusion of "I'm in this on my own, thanks" began to crumble on account of weakness and serious digestive problems, an accompanying feeling of shame at *being seen* began to become apparent. The ego loves to hide behind its masks of having it all together and being in control. When faced with the prospect of being seen running to the toilet halfway through a meditation session or not being able to get out of bed in the morning, it panicked. My initial response was to try to hide even more and make out like it was all deliberate in some way. It seemed safer if I could appear to be in control. So rather than admit that I hadn't slept and then crashed out at 4 A.M., I would instead concoct tales of how I had been meditating all night! Rather than ask for help when my stomach began to lose its capacity to digest certain foods, I pretended it was a deliberate ascetic practice. For a while I even managed to convince myself that this was the case—you can imagine the confused state of being that led to.

Trying to seal myself off from my own vulnerability was a disaster. Yet gradually the reality began to sink in: "Right now I feel ashamed. Right now I am embarrassed at being perceived of as weak. Right now I am scared of letting others in." Ironically, beginning to compassionately attend to these responses within myself was much less effort than trying to pretend everything was fine. That was a lot of work and yielded only bitter fruit. On the other hand, gently and sensitively exploring the wall between self and other—beginning to taste for myself what the *actual* results of opening to the help and support of my community were—began to reveal a whole new dimension of wonder, gratitude, and connection. As it turned out, this was the real medicine I needed—not just in the context of being ill but in the context of my whole life on this planet.

Around this time, I was very fortunate to have met my first teacher as a novice monk, Ajahn Viradhammo, whom I briefly mentioned earlier. It was in his presence that I first began to see what was really going on in myself: the tightness of my clinging to the illusion of independence. I also began to see the possibility of a different orientation altogether—one that was exemplified in his own relationship to the community we lived in. I mention him here to acknowledge that the process I am describing was not self-generated. It was on account of his example, which blew me right open and continues to be a source of deep inspiration to this day, that I began to realize the profound shift that can arise when we let down the walls of the heart and allow ourselves to be seen. Ajahn was and is an exceptional human being. If it wasn't for his presence, I am not sure how I would have survived those first few years of getting ill. The process could have gone down a whole different track. The power of his presence, to put it simply, lay in the complete absence of judgment, fixed interpretations, and stories about what was going on for me. What he offered was transparency of being and a tender, edgeless compassion. As I began to slowly open up about what was going on with my health, I was stunned by the absence of projections or even projects to "fix it" or make it all better. Instead I powerfully, palpably felt something I had never felt before—it is hard to describe, but it was like he was meeting me as if he *was* me and speaking from a place where there were no walls at all. There was only love—there was no inside or outside. I recall returning from a long trip away; Ajahn Viradhammo approached me with open arms inviting me in for a hug with the words "I missed you, brother." I was stunned. Not knowing what to say, I nervously received it. But something in me shifted. I recognized something I had been missing my whole life—the fact that in one way or another, I am always held. My time with Ajahn was a continual teaching in the power of connection and love, and I remain deeply indebted to him for this. The mirror of his unconditional love gradually began to educate my heart in the possibility of that same quality—for myself and for those around me. In the mirror of his complete absence of judgment, revulsion, or discomfort around what was happening to my body, I began to slowly find a way to reach out to others and to allow myself to be helped. Being in the presence of someone so loving and free of personal agenda showed me a new way of being in the world that was connected and open rather than sealed off.

Perhaps the most profound gift Ajahn Viradhammo shared with me was an openness about his own vulnerability and suffering. He didn't act like the everyday challenges of human life were unfamiliar or petty; rather, he was right there, resonating with all of it, within himself and in others. I can recall one striking example vividly. It was on a muggy spring afternoon on the day of an annual Buddhist festival. I had missed the meal and community gathering and was crashed out in my hut— exhausted, bloated, and in pain from the previous day's meal and weighed down by a cloud of depression and feelings of failure. In an attempt to keep the world out, I had drawn the curtains and lay in the half-light, brooding. Outside I heard a voice call out to me. My initial thought was, "Oh, no. Who's bothering me now? Go away," but I crawled to the curtain to peek outside anyway. There was Ajahn Viradhammo, waving and looking gently concerned. Having the abbot of a monastery visit you in the afternoon is not a common occurrence in the Thai Forest tradition, so it must have been important. I greeted my teacher and invited him in. As it turned out, he just wanted to see how I was doing. That in itself took me by surprise. It was so touching to realize that someone cared, and even more so that it was my teacher. As we began talking, I shared how I was doing and how despairing my mind had gotten. Ajahn seemed happy listening, so I began to open up more about what was going on. I found myself saying, "Sometimes I get caught in really dark thoughts. I know I would never follow them, but they do appear in flashes in my mind." When I said this I felt ashamed and a bit scared. It was the first time I had shared these thoughts with anyone. They seemed so personal and "bad" that I had locked them away whenever they came up. But somehow it felt good to express them in the safety of my teacher's presence. "Yeah, I have those too sometimes," replied Ajahn, contemplating his own heart. "It's normal. It's just the mind isn't it? The mind thinks all kinds of stuff. Especially in the middle of pain. Just don't follow them, eh?" The joy I felt was intense. For some reason I laughed out loud, in that way when you realize something so obvious that you hadn't noticed before and are caught in the awe of the moment. It wasn't "my" secret darkness—it was the human mind. And, hey, if my profound teacher had those thoughts sometimes, maybe I wasn't so flawed after all! Our conversation wove in and out of chuckling at the pathos of the human condition, listening to more serious reflections on the nature of the mind, and sharing spaces of silent reflection. By revealing his own vulnerability and humanizing those feelings and thoughts I felt were shameful and secret, my teacher invited me into the reality of our human connectedness, our shared experience, our mutuality. A big chunk of my inner wall came crashing down as the heart opened in celebration.

In the course of your life you may be fortunate enough to come across such people who open you up beyond what you thought was possible and offer you a space of trust in which to share your experience as it is, not as you think it should be. It could be a friend, a relative, a therapist, or a spiritual mentor. It is important to recognize such people when you meet them. Sometimes there may be initial feelings of fear and aversion that arise as your walls are challenged by their vulnerability. This is natural. However, rather than retreating back into a familiar state of being, it is important to remain open, to remain curious. Of course, this involves trust, and it takes time to discern the nature of a person's intentions. There is no hurry. The beauty of being in the presence of someone who models a new way of being for us is that it offers us, by way of a kind of osmosis, an example of what is possible. It offers us an invitation to do what is really needed—to find those self-same qualities in our own heart. The more we do that, the more we recognize the love that is already there in those who care for us, support us, and look out for our well-being. And the more we recognize it, the more it begins to flow.

Not all my experiences in relationship have been like the one I described above, though I count myself very lucky in terms of the many great people I have met in my life—my teachers, family, and friends. While it is very powerful to be in the presence of a deeply loving and awake human being, it is not a case of trying to find someone "out there" to save us. The heart of the practice is to learn the beauty of interdependence and surrender from the inside out regardless of the external circumstances or the quality of being folks are reflecting back at us. When we do this, the whole nature of relationship changes, and we find that the way others respond to us changes as well. There is a kind of magic in this. We see that there is in fact no fixed "them" and no fixed "me"—there is only relating in the moment. The experience of being cared for by other human beings can then become a practice in itself—it becomes the crucible for our inquiry, for exploring new ways of responding, and for tasting the joy and love that is present just under the surface of our meeting with another. Sometimes it is subtle—just a quiet, shared acknowledgement. Other times it is a celebration.

As we will see, though, there are cases or situations in which you will need to be prepared to exert your own capacity to say "no," to create a boundary, or to reduce your contact with someone. Allowing yourself to wholeheartedly receive the generosity of another is very different from situations where emotional abuse is involved or where unhealthy power dynamics are being perpetuated. Creating a healthy boundary is very different from being trapped behind a wall. On the deepest level we can find the capacity for equanimity or forgiveness in our hearts, yes. But on the relative level—especially in the context of the vulnerability that comes with illness—we also need to fully own our own inner strength, which is none other than the power of self-kindness in action.

BRINGING FORTH THE BEAUTIFUL

Realizing the power of the good heart has quite possibly saved my life. The beauty of having examples of true compassion and generosity mirrored back to me by my teachers and wise friends is that it awakened me to the profound power of this goodness. As a result, it has been a source of meaning and refuge during times of prolonged incapacity and limited ability to function in the world. We can often fall into states that obsess upon what we have lost, what we can no longer do, or all the ways our action is inhibited. I certainly can. When this happens, I find that something has been forgotten. It may be something we have forgotten for a very long time, but it is always right here, underneath the self-definitions of who we are and what we are able to do. It is the power to manifest the good heart in our interactions with others and bring beauty into the world. Please don't underestimate this. Accessing this potential can breathe freshness and meaning into difficult situations, long days in bed, or periods off work.

When we are ill, one powerful way we can consciously bring forth beauty and benefit to others is through our speech. Even though we can't help someone move house or surprise our partner by cleaning the garage, we always have the option of speaking in a way that conveys warmheartedness, love, and respect. I have found the conscious practice of kind, generous, or warmhearted speech to be a constant source of self-respect and confidence of heart in the face of physical limitations. In all Buddhist traditions, the practice of kind speech is held in high regard. We all know how much power speech has. A harsh comment can affect someone for weeks, even years. Our speech has the power to brighten someone's day or to sour it. Knowing this causal law, we don't have to leave it up to chance. Our awareness can attend to what we intend and what place in ourselves our speech is coming from before we actually say it. Once we get the feeling of how this works, kind speech can be a source of inner delight as well as a way of touching someone else's heart. Making others feel happy makes us happy. It's really quite a simple equation.

In exploring the ways we speak and training our attention to choose benevolence and warmheartedness, we may come across habits of cynicism or self-judgment in the process. It is normal to view such ways of speaking as either sycophantic, false, or too "nice." Those concepts of what kind speech is miss its real potential. Obviously we don't want to be fake about it—it is easy to tell when it is merely a posture rather than an expression of the open heart. But when it comes from our authentic presence, there is great power in kind speech. Making someone smile, complimenting something they have done, or letting them know how much we appreciate them brightens the moment and brings our own good heart alive. As we have already seen with the cultivation of loving-kindness, the good heart is the open heart. The open heart melts contracted states of fear and mistrust. A heart free of contraction is the foundation for the feeling sense of freedom in this moment. It is all connected.

Underlying the good heart is the feeling-intelligence of *harmlessness*. Although phrased in the negative, as the absence of something, it is a very potent template for investigating our inner intentions. If we act or speak out of the intention to harm others in coarse or subtle ways, our chances of healing the mind's tendencies toward *inner* harm in the form of self-criticism or guilt are very limited. We have already seen how much pain and limitation the mind of inner violence can cause us. It is the same, of course, with that intention directed externally. Through exploring wise and effective means of handling our inner turbulence, we realize that the shift requires something else in order to be effective: a commitment to stop making the stories connected to those turbulent energies a reality through our speech and action. It is natural to feel frustrated, angry, and irritated when we are ill. We can't control what will arise in our heart and mind when difficult conditions put the squeeze on us. What we do have a say over is whether or not we turn those energies into the intention to harm, lash out, or put down those around us. Making space around negative energies gives us this freedom. Through a sincere concern and curiosity about harm and harmlessness, we learn the secrets of healthy relationship. No one likes to feel like we mean them harm. Everyone loves to be regarded with respect and to feel safe in our presence. When we become skilled in the art of choosing what we want to offer to another person and what we want to work at letting go of, we begin to see and feel those self-same qualities manifest in those around us. Committing to non-harm is an essential support for transformation and well-being.

It is important to note here that in the Buddha's teaching on the mind, harmlessness refers to the quality of present-moment intention rather than trying to absolutely control the outcome of actions and speech or how they will be interpreted. It is not meant to set up an expectation that the chaotic nature of how others may perceive our intentions will change. However, attuning to the felt sense of intention is something powerful that we can do. Can you notice the feelings in your body when you intend harm? Do you notice a darkening or hardening when the volition to put someone down or cause them pain arises in you? What is that like? Try this exercise in embodied awareness for a few moments. Experiment with it. Get to know it. There's no need to feel guilty about it.

Now feel what it is like to remember the open heart, the good heart. How does it feel in the body when you wish for another person to be well? It is a very different quality, isn't it? The open heart recoils at the thought of harming another being. That is its nature. Treasuring and nurturing this heart intelligence in ourselves and aligning our intentions in relationship with it gradually awakens an inner strength. True harmlessness is a strength, not a weakness. When we trust that we don't want to cause pain to others, that trust allows us to be steadfast and strong in meeting those very impulses as they arise in the present moment. It is much harder to hold them with compassionate presence if we don't have this core commitment to harmlessness on the relational level. In fact, if we are merely acting them out, we can't see what they are at all.

THE GIVING IN RECEIVING

There is also a profound kind of offering that we can make when we wholeheartedly receive the kindness or help of another with an open heart. You may not have looked at it this way before, and there may in fact be certain stories that arise in you that suggest the opposite. This practice of direct awareness can make it possible to shine a light upon those stories within your mind. For example, you may experience stories of being a "burden" the moment your caregiver arrives and then unconsciously act out of that assumption, caught in a state of apology and guilt. This creates the wall we have been exploring above and also prevents you from experiencing the actual human connection that is taking place in the present moment. Wouldn't it feel much richer, more sacred, even, to be open to receive what is being offered, miraculously, from another human being and find a place in yourself that can celebrate that rather than feel ashamed about it? Receptivity is the key practice here. If you attune to that, even just as a concept, you will begin to see the ways your heart obstructs it in the present moment.

In order to receive, we have to be here. We have to be available, in this moment, to experience what is being offered to us by another. When we are lost in stories or hardened projections about either our own lack of worthiness or the irritation of having to have "this [insert adjective] person" come and do these things when we would rather just be alone and well again, then we are not here. We are in a fantasy. It may seem like reality, but in fact it is a fabricated state, conjured into being by the ever-creative wall-building faculty of our mind and heart. Seeing it as such is the beginning of a wonderful shift.

What kinds of walls do you notice in your own heart when it comes to relating to others from the vulnerable place of illness? Take some time to reflect on that. Use your memory creatively and see if you can gently contact whatever in you arises when others are offering assistance, when you are being seen, when you need to reach out and ask for help. Do this in an embodied way; really feel the response. Sense what it does in your belly or your chest. Can you feel if any of those reactions create a feeling of closing or tightening? Soften your grip around the sensations themselves, remembering that the heart of this practice is always a nonjudgmental awareness of whatever you uncover. Just allow yourself to resonate with those sensations. Be gentle, but also be clear. Don't get pulled into the stories that they try to suck your attention into. Stay with the feelings in your body, and feel for yourself where they come from and what they are saying. What do they assume about life? What do they *feel* about other people? Spend some time being intimate with those forces in your mind, heart, and body. Remember to be your own best friend in the process.

One thing that can be easy to forget when we are ill and in the presence of another's generosity is the blessing that we ourselves can offer them through the quality of *how* we receive what is being given. No human interaction is ever one way. There is always a mutuality, even if it remains unacknowledged. Rather than leaving this realm of mutual connection murky or infused with undercurrents of resistance and guilt, we can instead fully infuse it with our conscious intention and attention. This is wisdom in relationship. If you think back to a time when you have offered a gift to someone and they have wholeheartedly delighted in it—a time when you really felt that it meant something to them—how did that affect you? Can you sense how much richer the exchange of energy is when that happens? Using our memory in this way helps to understand how our response is affecting those who are offering us their time, support, or care. We can ask ourselves, "How would I like *them* to experience the interaction?" Inquiring in this way opens up a whole new possibility for joy and meaning in the midst of situations that may feel very uncomfortable for our ego-mind. It offers an opportunity to transform our way of perceiving and relating into one that creates a field of mutual appreciation and sharing rather than just being another predictable projection. In doing so the stories that give rise to these projections themselves lose their grip on the mind. They are seen more clearly for what they are. We feel the walls dissolve a little more every time we remember than we can connect and we can choose how we want to relate. Great wonder and delight can emerge whenever we do this. When we let in and communicate our appreciation for the help we receive, it makes *us* feel better. We have found meaning again, and it feels good. It also greatly enriches the experience of the person we are sharing the moment with. We find that we actually do have something to give, something to offer, in the midst of limitation and difficulty: our very own heart itself.

MIRRORS OF CAUSALITY

As we have seen in the examples above, it is possible to get to know causality in relationship and engage it in a positive and empowered way. We are very sensitive creatures and pick up upon the ways of being reflected back at us by those around us. It is a mirroring effect that is at the heart of the original teaching on relational *karma* in the early Buddhist discourses. This causal feedback loop can either reinforce the wall of separation and alienation (as well as the accompanying shadow states of guilt and self-criticism) or can gradually create a positive feedback loop of trust, mutuality, and an appreciation of the power of the open heart. When we respond to others with openness and receptivity, it gives them permission to do the same in themselves— it allows them access to their own inner wellspring of goodness and richness of heart where positive qualities can unfold in a space of trust. If we are negative, defensive, or closed up, there is less chance of this arising unless the other person is exceptional or has done a lot of spiritual or psychological work already.

When we inquire into the walls in our own heart and how own our responses affect first our own well-being and in return the attitudes and mind states of another person, whether it be a caregiver, spouse, or relative, we create an opportunity for both of us to be nourished. By making it easier and more enjoyable for others to offer support and assistance to us, physical or otherwise, the quality of their offering becomes richer as well. This in turn makes it easier for us to access our own openness, to relax into a sense of trust in the relationship, and to express our appreciation. The more we do this, the more this state of being is mirrored in the other, and their own experience of the relationship becomes richer. This happens both internally, in terms of the mind states they find themselves being able to access, and externally, in terms of the positive flow of their interactions with us. It is a win-win situation on the level of the heart, even in the midst of the loss and discomfort that comes with illness. It allows us to discover a happiness that is more intimate, direct, and sustainable than that of personal control over conditions, experiences, and even other people. It is the happiness that flows forth from the open heart itself. The good heart becomes a shared experience and gradually gathers its own power. When it does so, we find that it works miracles in the most unexpected and surprising of ways.

THE GRATITUDE CONNECTION

As we have seen, the mind has a very well-trained capacity to focus on what is "wrong" rather than what is OK, nonproblematic, or even very fortunate and blessed. This is true for both the physical self and our relationship to others. The human mind has an amazing knack for focusing on things about others that we don't like. We get stuck in our perceptions of "she always does . . ." or "he never says . . ." and begin relating to our cardboard cutout mental images of the other person rather than the ever-changing mystery that they are. This creates an unfortunate kind of tunnel vision in our awareness that blocks out an appreciation of the deeper reality taking place. We forget what it feels like to experience gratitude.

I should mention here, however, that using gratitude as a template for investigation and cultivation never means trying to whitewash experience and ignore how we actually feel about things. As with all areas of inquiry, it's always best to start from a place of vulnerability and self-honesty. From a connection to presence, self-kindness, and a spacious awareness of our internal states and feelings, we can begin to notice where our mind goes and what the results of that are. From this place—the place of reality—we have the ability to choose what to focus on and what to gently let go of. Rather than contracting and solidifying well-trodden pathways of criticism and fault-finding, we can instead explore a different option. We can attend to the miracle of human kindness—the blessing of being held by others—and allow that to affect us in a real, personal way. This is the birth of authentic gratitude.

Instead of applying a set of "shoulds" to our interactions with others (and then beat ourselves up with for not having manifested them), gratitude is actually a way of experiencing and sharing happiness and joy. It is not a way of saying "You shouldn't feel angry and embarrassed right now. Come on, feel grateful." That is a disaster. Instead, it begins with an interest in what is actually here, like all of the qualities and practices we have been exploring. If we feel closed off and embarrassed, for example, we can attend to that with a direct, compassionate presence, free of judgment. These are natural human feelings. Our awareness can span the sensations and resonate with them, feeling for where the energy is in the body, how it feels in the belly, the chest, or even the face.

When we have entered into the real, we are then in a position to attend to how we are perceiving the interaction with another person, whether it be in our bedroom, our home, or a hospital or doctor's office. We may then begin to notice that we primarily have been focusing on our own self-image—how we think we are being perceived—rather than being open to the presence of the other person, their expressions, their gestures, and their quality of being. The stories may be compelling and familiar, yet they create a wall in our human interactions. This wall arises from an instinctive need to protect ourselves, as we have seen, but in doing so it obstructs the ability to access a more vital and spontaneous response to the present moment. There is no need to judge it, however. We can just acknowledge it gently and include this wall in our spacious, embodied presence as well.

From this place, a shift can occur. The spark that ignites it is our own conscious choice to see, feel, and receive the deeper meaning of what is happening underneath the stories and protective mechanisms of the mind and heart. Of course, if it is a situation where there is a real problem or we are uncertain about whether we can trust the person who is attending to us, then it is not the right time for gratitude. It is the time for boundaries and clarity, as we will see. But if the situation is what seems like a run-of-the-mill interaction, we shift our attention in this way, relaxing the wall of fixed perceptions around ourselves and the other person and allowing what is actually here to touch the heart.

Stepping back from the stories and self-images of the mind, we can open into a sense of appreciation for the care we are being offered right now. When we do this, it simultaneously expands our capacity to receive the other person with a whole-hearted presence. We can begin to notice the larger human context that is here—the connection taking place through the offering of a gentle touch, a kind word, assistance with taking medicines, a cup of tea, or a simple checking in. We can be here for it rather than lost in our perceptions, interpretations, and habitual reactions. Being here with the connection and kindness we are being offered automatically opens the heart into a feeling of gratitude and thankfulness. We don't have to force it into being—it arises from touching the reality of human goodness in the present moment. When it is present it feels pleasant, uplifting, and refreshing. It gives the moment meaning. Rather than feeling like a chore or a spiritual identity to prop up, authentic gratitude fills the heart with a reason to be glad, a reason to celebrate. When we are exhausted in bed or navigating hours of discomfort, incapacity, and pain, any reason to celebrate is a blessing. And what better reason than a recognition of the miracle of being held, of being cared for, of being loved? This quiet kind of celebration fills us up from the inside out.

When you have experimented a little with this new way of being in relationship in the present moment, it will begin to occur to you that there have in fact been many such moments of kindness you have received over the course of your life that you have never really taken into your heart. You may realize that in fact your life has been woven from all these threads of support and nourishment from others, from the subtle to the profound. What is it that makes you who you are? What is it that allows you to keep going? What gave you the confidence to pick up this book? It is very hard to separate nature from nurture when we really begin to reflect on our lives. All the kind words we have received, the phone calls, the offerings of support, going right back to the food and lodging that most of us received from our parents. In fact, it is impossible to remember every moment of generosity and kindness we have received in our lives. When we open to this fact, a feeling of awe and wonder suffuses the heart. It is the awe of the thankful heart. It is gratitude for the fact of having been held by this human web ever since we were born.

Once again, it must be said that this is not an invitation to pretend there hasn't been pain, loss, and disappointment on the relational level. Rather, it is a way of opening us up to a reality that is simultaneously true. There is always the bright, the good, the blessed. We don't need to reflect much to remember the pain and the hurt. What we are not so good at is remembering all of the gifts we have received. Directing our attention in this way opens up a whole world of new possibilities in our relationship to others.

Shortly after the experience of hitting the wall of hunger and exhaustion in the monastic setting, I went through a period of facing the walled-off phenomenon of embarrassment and shame in my own heart. Turbulent as it was, it finally led to the possibility of opening into a newfound feeling of gratitude for the fact of being held and supported by the kindness of my community. As I mentioned earlier, the monastic form I was in was very strict, particularly around one's personal control around food. For better or for worse, there are no official exceptions or provisions for a special diet, even if it arises out of physical illness. To be offered this possibility was and is a very rare occurrence within the Thai Forest tradition, which functions primarily through the generosity of the Buddhist community and the capacity of the monks to accept whatever is offered. As it became clear that the only way I could keep going was to eat a special restricted variety of foods, I began to feel like a failure. I imagined that the other monks viewed me in all sorts of negative ways—breaking from the tradition, being weak, or just being an annoyance in some way. In retrospect, I am sure most of this was a construction of my mind (though I am sure some of it was true for people some of the time!). What also pushed an old button for me was all the extra work that the community would be undertaking on my account. Perhaps it has something to do with being born in the United Kingdom, but "not making a fuss" is something hardwired into the rules of my ego-mind. And there I was, not only making a fuss but having people change their routines and make extra efforts to help me. I was overcome with shame and guilt, imagining the other monks whispering in private corners, "*Tsk tsk.* Look at him. How selfish." My whole being curdled with feelings of embarrassment, inadequacy, and the wish to just hide somewhere and not be seen. But there I was.

When it came time for me to walk in the line of monks to collect my daily meal off the "special" tray each day, I became aware of the welling up of perceptions and feelings of "wrongness" in my whole body and mind. I could feel my face flush with the sense of being looked at. The storytelling mind kicked in and began to fixate upon notions of how I felt I was being viewed; as a result, mealtimes were experienced as a combination of physical relief and emotional turmoil. In search of respite from this mind-made suffering, I fell back on the seemingly endless patience and support of Ajahn Passano and Ajahn Amaro, my teachers at this time, who kindly and gently reassured me that indeed I was making all this stuff up. It took many conversations to come round to believing them, but checking in with the *actual* reality as a contrast to the internal perceptions of "them" that would assail me throughout the process of receiving and eating the new diet provided an important touchstone. It invited me to question why I was so hell-bent on torturing myself at a time when so much was being offered by such kind folks to support my very survival.

Thankfully, the capacity to question the mind's projected ideas of a disapproving "them" and a flawed and weak "me" grew as each day passed. Having no choice but to face the mind and its narratives squarely as mealtimes came around was in many ways a gift. While I wanted to run away and hide, instead I had to find a way to turn the situation around—right there in the midst of the heightened self-consciousness that came from being cared for in such conspicuous ways. Once we had gotten our food, we would return to the hall where we sat quietly in meditation while the abbots chatted with the folks who offered the food. On one such occasion as I was sitting quietly, waiting to dive into my lentils and tofu, I found myself bringing to mind the face of the kind person who spent extra time preparing my meal. A feeling of warmth and richness spontaneously began to fill my heart. I found myself breaking into a little smile. It wasn't a contrived effort to feel grateful; this feeling of happiness arose just through attending to the other person—through opening to the reality of their generosity. It was quite simple. All of a sudden I realized the tragedy of my attitude. As if waking from a bizarre dream, it dawned on me, "Dude. That's insane. Here you are, being supported by such grand-hearted human beings, and you're still focusing on what might be 'bad' about it all!" Marveling at the insanity of my own mind, I consciously began to bring to mind more and more people who were involved—the guests helping in the kitchen, my brother monks, and one friend of the monastery who drove three and a half hours from San Francisco, often with extra goodies to prevent me from starving. Really allowing this into the heart for the first time, free of shame and the effort to prop up an image of being strong or capable on my own, felt like opening the door to a reservoir of fullness and happiness that had always been there. I had just been avoiding it like crazy. In fact, I realized that I had inadvertently been hiding from the full scope of human connectedness. Part of my awareness was subconsciously afraid of the power of that. Letting myself take it in, however, wasn't frightening or overpowering at all—it was an experience of release. Awareness was released from the constricting prison of self-obsession. It opened into a reality that took the heart beyond the personal and into the feeling of being held by a living, loving web of connectedness that was already there. The meal that day was delicious.

The quality that arose in that space before eating my meal is akin to something the Buddha described as one of the four qualities of the open heart, alongside kindness, compassion, and equanimity. This heart resonance, *mudita* in the Pali language, has often been translated as "empathetic joy." It arises when we attend to the positive, bright, or profound qualities in other people rather than our own internal dramas. This kind of attention is a portal into the connectedness we have been exploring above and the accompanying potential to feel the simple happiness of mutual appreciation. In this way it is very close to the quality of gratitude. When the goodness we are attending to in another person is directed toward ourselves, gratitude arises automatically. Being thankful is a natural movement in our human being. We don't have to make it up or try to force it into existence. Through making ourselves available to receive everyday kindness or simple acts of caring from our partner, our friends, and our caregivers, the subjective experience of the present moment becomes one of quiet thankfulness. This thankfulness expresses itself as love in our speech and our actions. Attending in this way is far more healing to our entire system than being caught within the walls of separation spawned by the ego-mind. It is medicine for the heart.

EMPOWERED OPENNESS

There will be times, however, when gratitude and receptivity to the goodness of another is not what is being asked for. Not everyone you come into contact with will be engaged in freely giving and offering you kindness. Most of you will know viscerally and painfully what it is like to be in the presence of someone who is caught in a mask of condescension or harshness. These kinds of experiences can be both disturbing on the level of being and disastrous on the practical level if we become enmeshed in perceptions and beliefs held by the other person.

Going to see a professional for advice, for example, puts us in a very vulnerable position already. When we are weak or rundown, we are more susceptible to conceding to unhealthy power dynamics and saying yes to something we are in actual fact not sure about at all. So we need to remember that being open doesn't mean being weak. As we have seen earlier with the balance of kindness and equanimity, finding our ground in awareness and the open heart means having access to the whole experience of our humanness—not just a two-dimensional spiritual ideal of being "nice." Sometimes you have to stand firm and refuse to be caught in the projections of another—whether it be a doctor, a relative, or a loved one. The wisdom that arises when we enter into the directness of pure presence is that which refuses to buy into fixed views of what is going on—either our own or those of others. Over time, this wisdom develops antibodies that seek out and detect the toxins of judgment and negativity. As we become more sensitive, we are able to feel these more acutely. And we know directly that they only bring suffering and have the potential to make the condition of the body much worse.

Refusing to get caught in the judgments or dismissiveness of another person doesn't mean being closed off to advice, however. In relationship, the Middle Way also applies. It can manifest as an ability to discern where particular advice is coming from in another person and how we are picking it up in ourselves. Sometimes the advice we are being offered is coming from a genuinely caring place in another and we pick it up with self-judgment and turn it into feelings of shame. I have done this on many occasions. In this case, awareness can trust the intuition of the goodness of the other person's intentions and compassionately hold our own painful response. At other times we can sense that advice is arising from a mind state in the other person that isn't so positive or perhaps is exclusively focused on fixing or changing us without an acceptance of what is actually here. I am sure many of you will have experienced this in the course of your illness. This kind of attitude unfortunately can be infectious and has the power to take us away from our own openness to the facts of the present moment if it goes unnoticed and unchecked in our own mind and heart. When we lose the qualities of acceptance and self-compassion, we are more susceptible to becoming divided in ourselves with an attitude of rejection or desperate seeking once again. Often both of these dissociative reactions will occur simultaneously—they are two sides of the same contracted state. So being in the presence of someone who is clinging to the idea of "You must be fixed. Your condition is unacceptable. You need to be healed" is an occasion to put up a red flag in awareness and be very careful. Trusting your own readout of where another person is coming from through noticing the tone of their voice or the look in their eyes, for example, will save you from becoming enmeshed in their mind states of rejection and division—if you stay present and true to what you value in yourself.

On other occasions, we sense unhealthy power dynamics at work. This can often manifest as a feeling that the other person always needs to be "right," for example. While this may be true on a relative level, if we can sense that the person is clinging too tightly to this conviction and isn't allowing any space for listening, inquiry, or genuine understanding of what we are experiencing, then something in us knows that this isn't a good relationship to just give in to. We need to stand firm, but without losing our openness in the process. There are also those times when we think we should trust someone, even though we don't, and beat ourselves up for not trusting them (although something deeper in us knows we probably shouldn't). It just doesn't feel right. This can be very confusing. In such cases it is useful to keep feeling things out with a sense of curiosity. In the end we may not know why the relationship doesn't feel right, but we can honor our own feelings and needs. We don't have to know for sure that our intuition is right. But we can trust that our intention is to take care of our own mind, heart, and body. Following this intention never brings bad results. It may mean that we need to ask questions, to get to know the other person more. Or it may mean that it is time to allow things to naturally fade out. If these decisions come from our own connection to the present-moment dynamics of our engagement, we are less likely to second-guess ourselves in hindsight. We trust ourselves.

NOT-KNOWING, FULLY SENSING

Arriving at this kind of trust in relationship requires the capacity to rest with a degree of not-knowing. In the same way that we can learn to unhook from the internal stories and projections we have around illness when we are alone and in discomfort or pain, we can learn to see through the stories of self and other our mind generates while in the presence of another person. Trusting in this unknowing can feel disorienting at first, so it is important to feel grounded in the practice of awareness with regard to your own mind states first. This may take a while to get used to. If what I describe below sounds beyond your abilities or confusing right now, then feel free to put it aside until you feel ready.

As with the practice of awareness on the internal level, exercising the capacity for an open, clear awareness while in the presence of another requires seeing with our own eyes. Pure awareness is always utterly simple and uncomplicated. It isn't a perception, an interpretation, a measurement, or a judgment. It is the fact of being aware itself. Seeing with our own eyes means choosing to empower this faculty of awareness and to feel ourselves *as it*. The mind is habituated to moving out of this ground through a desire to understand or know using a story, a narrative of some kind. While this kind of knowing can have uses and an accuracy to it, it often serves to obscure a more direct readout of the moment—one that is sensed when awareness releases its grip on rigid, fixed thought formations. Trusting that we can do this while in the middle of a conversation or listening to another person talking to us, for example, is a radical act and can feel both dangerous and liberating. But it is only dangerous to the mind that is addicted to its own repetitive structures of interpreting the moment. To our true being it is pure refreshment, like waking up anew to a wonder and vitality that had previously been hidden.

You may notice that when another person is talking to you, you are often only half there. You see them, hear them, and understand the words they are saying, but your mind is also engaged in an inner dialogue. You are wishing they would stop talking or saying, in your mind's eye, "Here he goes again." Or you are holding back from really being there through perceptual filters of "You don't understand me," or the opposite, "You have all the answers. I can't trust myself." Such internal voices often arise out of filters in the mind that are nonverbal, but are present in the form of more subtle walls in the mind and heart. They are mind-made masks that we take to be a real "me" or a real "you" and become stuck within. But reality is always far more ambiguous. In fact, it is just the experience of seeing, hearing, feeling, and sensing. The way through this labyrinth of walls and masks is the way of unknowing.

When you are in the middle of a conversation, for example, you can ask yourself, "What is it like to just listen and create space around what is being said? What is it like to consciously relax all the mind's grasping at words and ideas and instead allow awareness to receive the fact of the other person in the present moment?" This reestablishes our attention in awareness itself and quickens our capacity to be here for experience as it is.

Be aware of the other person. Here they are, in front of you. Notice the color of their face, their clothes, their hair. Hear the tone of their voice. Notice their eyes. Actually seeing and hearing consciously like this helps awareness release itself from the grip of narratives and perceptions that may be assaulting the mind in the moment. Once you have returned to this direct sensory experience, see if you can expand awareness a little more, so that now you are seeing and feeling the other person as a unified field in awareness.

The example the Buddha gave was of the method of stretching out a bull's hide that was used for leather in ancient India. Initially you would have this messy wrinkled thing in front of you. But you would clip it to pegs and use a wooden machine to stretch it out until all the wrinkles, crevices, and the shadowy areas disappeared. You could perceive it as a whole. I have always found this analogy useful in relationship. It is like unwrinkling awareness while in the presence of another human being. Rather than being a cue to dissociate, it is the ground of simplicity from which we can connect to our actual heart presence in the moment. When the mind is freed from all the extra proliferating and spinning that comes through reaction, habitual self-stories, and fixed perceptions of "her" or "him," we can actually attend to how the interaction is affecting us. We have created the space to return to the direct bodily sense of our response and can use the steadfastness of equanimity and the receptivity of self-kindness and compassion to really feel how their words and presence affect us. It is all right to be affected. It is being human. How we relate to this, however, determines how we will relate to the person we are talking to. When we can contact the feelings that are arising in this way, we are also in the right space to make decisions. Our intuition may be that a boundary is needed and we need to say "No" or "This isn't the right time." At other times, and with certain people in our lives, it may be right to share how we are being affected in a kind but strong way. Or we may feel a sense of trust and ease, and speak words that convey this quality, inviting the same feelings to arise in the other. Other times we may just remain quiet, listening, not-knowing, but fully present. The difference between this way of relating and our "normal" mode of being caught in internal voices, concocting viewpoints, reacting to things said, defending, or attacking is in the quality of presence itself. Allowing presence to unfold through first a willingness to un-know all of the mind's perceptual overlays and then return to the direct embodied experience of the relationship, we contact a deeper heart-wisdom that is responding from the freshness of the moment. From this place we are more able to set healthy boundaries and to act out of an inner strength that knows how to take care of ourselves. And of course we are also more available to be present for the goodness and kindness we are being offered and to offer it in return. The power and love of the open heart become available to us.

MEDITATION ON AWAKENING GRATITUDE

Take some time to settle into a posture that feels comfortable for you. It may be resting in a seat, lying down comfortably on your bed, or sitting on a cushion on the floor if your energy permits. Remember that the posture is secondary; it is your heart presence and sincerity of intention that really counts.

Take a few moments now to close your eyes and reconnect with the feeling-presence of your body. Be soft and loving with your attention. There is no need to force or strain. Instead, allow your genuine curiosity and wonder to give life to awareness itself. Rest as simple presence, breathing through your body with an intimacy and kindness toward the sensations you meet. Open your eyes and come back to these words when it feels right.

Now use the quality of wise attention and spacious awareness you have been cultivating to remember that mental stories are just so. They are being created in this moment. Remember that you can choose what you want to focus on. You don't have to remain in the spin of murky narratives. Your attention is your own.

With this in mind, feel what it is like to gently begin to bring to mind one kind act that someone has offered you recently—

one act that touched your heart and brought a feeling of being cared for. There is no need for it to be the "right one"—any one will do. Now with your eyes closed or open, feel what it is like to really let yourself be affected by that memory. Consciously relive it. Relive it many times in this moment. Feel how it feels. Really let it suffuse your heart. Bathe in the feelings that it brings up. Allow your human heart to celebrate that feeling of being regarded with love, generosity, or concern.

If the heart feels numb or a sense of "So what?" don't judge yourself or feel like it isn't working. You have all the time in the world. Keep using your attention to remember something that touched your heart—something you feel grateful for. It can be something very small, such as a smile or a kind word. Or something life-saving. The aim here is to allow yourself to be vulnerable to the goodness of another, to let it in. Be undefended in your whole body and mind as you do this. No one is watching. You can let down your guard. It is safe to let the flower of thankfulness bloom in your heart. Feel the life-giving power of that capacity you have. Let it restore and heal your sense of connection to the other humans you share this planet with. Let it blow out the cobwebs of mistrust from your being. Let it become a light that warms your whole being from the inside out. Play with wonderful possibility for as long as your energy allows.

8

Relating to Pain

NOBODY LIKES BEING in physical pain. I don't like it at all. I
can honestly say that after almost two decades of committed
meditation practice, I dislike being in pain as much as I ever did.
For many years I tried to become somebody who was always
equanimous with pain, but gradually the realization dawned on
me that this is actually a futile endeavor. My personality doesn't
like, want, or enjoy pain. Thankfully, however, this isn't the
point. The aim isn't to try to become somebody who likes pain
or doesn't feel aversion, dejection, fear, or desperation when it
arises. In this journey of finding freedom of awareness and peace
in our hearts, the aim is to become curious about those very reactions themselves. We don't have to like pain to understand it.
Instead, it is possible to investigate the nature of pain, our own
emotional reactions to it, and to shine the light of wisdom and
self-compassion onto our present-moment experience of the
phenomenon itself. Whenever we do this with sincerity, the existential suffering that usually accompanies the physical sensations begins to abate. We still may not like or want the experience

on a personal level, but our hearts don't have to close down in its presence. This is where our real freedom lies.

The nature of our human condition is to spend most of our lives trying to avoid pain, prevent it from arising, and distance ourselves from it. Yet, in some form or another, it persists. Our human bodies are vulnerable to pain. When they become ill, feelings of physical pain and discomfort generally accompany the experience. While it is possible (and often practical) to take steps to alleviate the intensity of the experience, at some point or another we will have no choice but to ask, "What is this pain I don't want, anyway?" The only way to answer that question is to look, feel, and sense deeply into the direct present-moment experience. Whenever we do this, we begin to see the experience of pain or discomfort with fresh eyes. In my own journey of relating to pain, I have found that there are in fact many powerful perspectives and practices that open us up to this fresh way of seeing and feeling.

IS PAIN THE SAME AS SUFFERING?

In all Buddhist teachings, there is a clear distinction between painful feeling and existential suffering. Although there is a very close causal relationship between them on the moment-to-moment level of our human mind and heart, in actuality they are not intrinsically entwined on the most fundamental level. Put simply, these teachings assert that it is possible to have an open heart while in the midst of unpleasant or painful sensations. Even though the causal progression from physical pain to emotional pain is often very quick and occurs underneath the radar of our awareness, it is possible to unhook and relax the emotional reaction from the actual physical sensation. In practical terms, this usually means softening and opening the contraction around pain and finding a place of refuge in the OK-ness of presence itself.

This perspective remains a very optimistic one for me personally. It points to a freedom that can be experienced right in the middle of the experience of the body, just as it is, and provides a mirror for all the ways the heart and mind equate painful feeling with suffering. However, it is important not to pick this invitation up as an ideal to be clung to and then try to grit our teeth and not suffer. Our habits of emotional suffering in the presence of physical pain are not resolved through trying to squeeze ourselves into a spiritual (or even "tough") persona of some kind. In fact, that kind of approach usually leads to an inner violence that results in the loss of the qualities of kindness and embodied compassion that we have been exploring. So part of this approach involves being vulnerable to how our heart contracts when pain arises and what stories the thinking mind begins to weave based on that contraction. As with all of these practices, the aim is to be like an explorer, scientist, or adventurer. We are courageously yet gently charting new territories in our being in order to understand how things actually are. It is only through this intimacy and honesty that we can begin to forge new ways of relating to physical pain. In my experience, often what is needed is a compassionate holding of the heart's suffering in its presence and a letting go of everything in the mind that wants to make something, anything, out of it. When nothing is made out of it, the pain changes from being a concept such as "this awful thing" to a dynamic field of sensations. We can work with that.

GETTING CLEAR ABOUT WHAT IS HERE

In the discourses of the Buddha there is a very handy framework designed to help us get some perspective on painful bodily sensations as phenomena in and of themselves. Given that people who lived and worked in northern India around 600 B.C. probably were far more vulnerable to extreme conditions on the physical level than we are today, working with sensation directly must have been a necessity. In many ways, living with chronic illness puts us in a similar position. When not even the comforts and conveniences of modern life can shield us from unwanted physical sensations, we need to find a way of meeting them as they actually are rather than what we want them to be or wish we could feel instead. In these early texts there are three different categories of sensation that all experiences of bodily feeling can be said to fall into: painful, pleasant, and neutral. It is important to note that the Pali word for sensation here, *vedana,* isn't referring to the emotional resonance that often accompanies it. It refers to the pure sensations that we can contact with awareness through using the direct experience of the body as our foundation for mindful presence. Can you sense the difference between those three kinds of sensation?

NEUTRAL SENSATION

The neutral sensations are the hardest to bring into awareness, yet they are the ones that are always here. We tend to overlook them, screen them out as non-events, or ignore them, but attending to the field of neutral sensations is a way of connecting to the body as a whole. It also provides a contrast and context for the other two kinds of sensations. You may have already become aware of this category of feeling when you explored the body scan meditation in chapter 2. Did you find yourself becoming aware of a whole field of previously unnoticed sensations just through the act of giving them attention? Remember what that was like. That is neutral bodily sensation. Part of the power of using the direct experience of the body as our foundation for meditation is that it strengthens this resource in neutral feeling and turns it into a potent aliveness. When we have a grounding in presence felt through bodily sensations, we have the strength to get some perspective on the other two kinds of feeling.

PLEASANT SENSATION

We all want pleasant sensations. They make us feel alive, can shift our mood, and have the power to reconnect us to a sense of optimism if we relate to them from a wise and aware place in ourselves. Yet when we cling to them or try to make them personal possessions, they paradoxically evade our grasp. Their subsequent loss then becomes the source of suffering. How often have you allowed yourself to experience a pleasant sensation such as the warmth of a hot bath or the feeling of sun on your face as *just that?* Do you notice the mind's tendency to subtly contract around it and grasp for more of that experience? What is pleasant feeling like when it is felt, enjoyed, and experienced without the need to grasp it, prolong it, or fabricate stories of yourself around it? Even seemingly benign stories such as *"Ah,* I wish it were like this forever. This is how it should be" can set us up for the pain of the divided heart. If we begin to associate a "good me" with pleasant sensation, weaving stories like "I'm back. This is who I really am. Who I really am feels this way," it conditions the future arising of despair, confusion, and self-aversion when those feelings naturally pass. We forget that we actually never left—we are always who we are. Pure presence doesn't need particular conditions in order to know itself. It just is, always. So exploring our relationship to pleasant feeling is part of becoming wise in the midst of physical pain. The two go hand in hand. Transforming our relationship to pleasurable physical sensation from one of clinging and identification into a deeper kind of open, grateful appreciation develops our capacity to remain steadfast and aware in the face of unpleasant feeling.

When we know that sensations are of the nature to change, the appearance of pain is far less of a surprise.

UNPLEASANT SENSATION

Can you notice the difference between unpleasant sensations such as throbbing, aching, pulsing, or burning in themselves and the meaning the heart and mind give them in the present moment? What is an unpleasant sensation when the perceptions and stories around what it means or how it will "never go away" are relaxed and seen through? What is the pure sensation like? These are the kinds of questions that are worth asking when you are experiencing physical pain. They are meant to point you directly back to the experience itself—to get a handle on just what it is that we are referring to when we talk about "pain." When we gently and compassionately delve underneath the layers of mental construction and heart contraction that come between the physical sensations and our awareness itself, we finally begin to meet painful bodily feeling as it is. This in itself is a radical shift.

In this third category of sensation, the words *pain* and *unpleasantness* are interchangeable. When you reflect on all the kinds of physical feeling that don't fall into the category of pleasant or just neutral, you will become aware that there are many different flavors of unpleasant feeling that you can experience in your body and that are heightened during the experience of illness. There can be a wide variety of experiences that are unpleasant on a physical level, from sharp pain to all-encompassing discomfort. The skill of awareness is to contact these sensations directly and know them as such. We can know "This is unpleasant right now. This is painful." Just knowing that clearly and directly helps us find clarity underneath all the extra layers of meaning the heart and mind inevitably spin around the experience—particularly in the moments when neutral or pleasant feeling give way to unpleasantness. Whether it is a heavy feeling of exhaustion, a tight feeling of constriction, a persistent headache, or a stabbing, localized sensation, we can know that it is *just so*. This clarity then allows us to pan out and broaden our perspective on the stories that are arising in the heart and the mind. We can also begin to sense how they interact with the sensations themselves and make unpleasantness much more unpleasant.

You may be wondering whether it is possible to just change our stories about pain—to tell ourselves that physical pain isn't so bad, or even flip around the perceptions from disliking to liking. Of course, our present-moment contemplations require a shift in the fundamental narrative we are giving our attention to. We can use narratives that are skillful to reorient the mind toward awareness and the open heart. These put us in the right place to explore our reactions to the pain or unpleasantness that is here. However, if our attention remains embedded in the storytelling mind, we miss out on the chance to really contact and understand what the sensations are in and of themselves. We can also strengthen a habit of denial or forced positivity in the face of experiences that, if we are honest, we neither want nor like. The path offered in this chapter is the direct one. It is also the most compassionate one. It is a way of relating to physical experience that doesn't depend on being positive all the time or trying to fix the mind into a rigid set of spiritual views about the pain that is arising. In my own experience, those strategies are extensions of the divided heart—the ego-mind that seeks to control experience, often at the expense of being vulnerable to the reality of the present moment as it actually is. Most of us who have lived with physical illness for any length of time come to a point where these strategies are no longer possible. The energy of division just runs out. What we are left with is the pure experience. While this can seem like a failure and bring up feelings of fear or self-blame at first, I would like to suggest that this failure to "like" the body's pain, make it special in some way, or even cover it over with spiritual perceptions is actually the start of the heart's real journey into well-being.

COMPASSIONATE CURIOSITY

Having gotten clear about what unpleasant sensation actually is in and of itself, we now come to the most important part—how to relate to it in the present moment. The magic of meeting pain or discomfort as it is (without the usual overlay of our stories about what it means) is that we are in the position to transform the primary relationship we have to it. We can't do this from our heads. This can only take place in the direct, embodied awareness we have already been cultivating. Our habitual response is to react to pain. There is a kind of retracting or flinching that happens when painful sensation arises. Awareness recoils and contracts from the sensation itself and inhabits a perception of what it *means* instead. These perceptions are often subconscious but can be gently unpacked in the light of mindful presence. We may have built these perceptions up over a lifetime; they are the subjective emotional tones that the mind very easily believes is the unpleasant feeling itself. However, in this practice of direct awareness, we begin to see that they are actually something extra that we are doing right now.

Of course there may be times when the painful sensations are too intense to be met with this kind of directness. Please honor that in yourself. This is not an encouragement to try to push yourself into a state of being that is going to be draining or emotionally taxing. If you feel like that is the case, I would encourage you to skip this chapter and perhaps return to focusing on the heart qualities of self-kindness and compassion rather than reading further and feeling guilty that you can't apply your attention. If energy isn't here, it isn't here. Acknowledging this takes humility, but it is also a deep expression of freedom and love for yourself. You are exercising your freedom to choose how and when you want to attend to the phenomena that accompany illness. You are trusting in the wisdom of kindness. This is always to be celebrated.

However, often your awareness will still have the capacity to meet how you *feel* about the pain. What is being called for in these times is a compassionate relationship to the emotional tone of heart that is arising in the moment. When we don't have the capacity, energy, or strength of mind, the thought of making painful sensation the primary focus of attention is altogether unappealing. So it is OK to acknowledge that and instead allow our awareness to inquire into the secondary level of what the pain appears to mean right now and how we *feel* about that meaning. This is the open heart in action. Even if awareness remains walled off from the unpleasantness arising in the present moment, you can relate to the raw energy of the heart just as it is. For example, if you have a splitting headache and need to lie down, you can just lie down. You may not have the capacity to attend to the unpleasantness of the sensations in your head—the piercing, throbbing pain—but you can gently give your attention to the emotions and accompanying perceptions that are arising in the present moment. You can hold yourself in a field of great kindness. Awareness can relax and soften around the very sense of "being here with this intense headache" right now. How does that feel in your heart? Is there an accompanying sense of self that arises, such as "I'm trapped" or "I'm being attacked"? Let awareness become interested in that very sense. Or the emotional reaction could be in response to the headache itself —our attention often configures painful sensation as an object that is bad or means us harm in some way, and then enters into a relationship of conflict with it. However, you can become aware of that too and feel into the primary currents of energy arising in the moment. How do they feel? What do they believe? Most important, what do they *do* to the painful feeling itself?

RELAXING AROUND PAINFUL SENSATION

If our awareness is completely identified with the perceptions and emotions that arise in response to painful sensation, it is likely that the sensations themselves will be begin to feel worse. Have you noticed that if you have feelings of enmity or anger toward pain, the painfulness increases? Many of the habitual reactions we have in response to pain or unpleasantness on the bodily level can make the sensations more pronounced. Fear and despair can have the same effect, as does anxiety about the future. Any kind of contraction around painful sensation inhibits relaxation and ease in the field of our bodily presence. We lose space. The result is that our attention clamps onto the pain and amplifies it. So relaxing our grip on those reactive mind states themselves—questioning and unfolding the apparent reality of what they want us to believe—is a potent way of alleviating the here-and-now intensity of the sensation that is present.

Often the core of our reaction will be a primal contraction of "no" around the pain. This "no" attempts to push it away from awareness but paradoxically makes a feature of it at the same time. This response is instinctual and natural; it doesn't need to be judged. However, if our awareness can meet the felt sense of this "no" with compassion and curiosity, it can have an effect of decreasing the intensity of the pain. Rather than feeling that we have to get rid of the impulse in our heart, body, and mind, we can become interested in it. What is it anyway? What does it want to protect? What is it afraid of? These are questions to take into your intuitive awareness rather than over-analyze. You can feel for the answers, which will always be unique to the changing landscape of the present moment. When you listen deeply in this way, the sense that pain is an enemy softens and fades. While the pain may still be there, something in the core of your being has relaxed and unbound itself from the extra layers of reaction and perception. There is a great feeling of relief and peace that accompanies this. Over time you may begin to notice certain patterns that your mind and heart gravitate toward, but the inquiry needs to be fresh, direct, and innocent if it is to really bring about a shift. This kind of shift doesn't come about through ego-driven willpower but through relaxing and softening around whatever is here while standing firm in the clarity of awareness.

One of the most powerful experiences I have had of this type of shift was about a year after I chose to leave the Buddhist monastic lifestyle. Unfortunately, my last few months as a monk had been accompanied by a full-body experience of severe eczema. When this phenomenon re-arose (which is often part of the life cycle of eczema, according to dermatologists) it was as bad, if not worse, than it had ever been. The entire surface of my body was purple, raw, and weeping lymph fluid twenty-four hours a day. It was as close to a physical hell as I have ever been in my life. After leaving the monastic lifestyle in order to take care of my body in a way more suitable to its needs, the intensity of the eczema continued. Very often I found myself up late at night, sleepless, wired, and in pain. It was after one such night that I found myself lying on the floor of my bedroom with my eyes closed, consumed by fear of the future and disaster stories of where my life was going. I could see the mind and heart spiraling into deeper states of despair. Life seemed like a nightmare.

At the bottom of this spiral, however, a voice arose in my heart and asked, "What's the problem right now?" The momentum of thought stopped. Awareness fell back into the present moment, relaxing and softening around the feelings and sensations that were actually there. The inner voice asked, "What if there is no problem with any of this?" Fragments of stories burst forth in fits and starts: "But you'll never be able to . . ." "This will never go away . . ." "This is bullshit . . ." and yet each time they arose, awareness met them with a clarity that saw them as thoughts fabricated in the present moment itself. The heart relaxed. The stories faded. Awareness then began to feel underneath the sense of time and the fixed view of "me and my life" and discovered a contracted knot of dark feelings in the pit of my stomach. After attending to it in the space of my own compassionate presence for a few minutes, the knot came alive and began to speak. "This is unfair," it said. For a few moments I just let myself rest with the sadness and heaviness of that feeling from a place of compassion for the whole predicament. That felt good—it felt more real than any story about the future or past or about "Who I will always be."

But then another, deeper intuition arose, to my surprise. It asked, "What if this moment is already perfect? What if you stop believing it's wrong?" In that moment the contracted state opened into a cool sense of relief and peace deep in my being itself. A smile arose for no reason, as feelings of a newfound freedom flooded the mind, the heart, and even the body. With a silent, curious mind, I got up, not bothering to change from my ragged sleep clothes, and walked outside. It was a beautiful summer's day. My senses felt alive despite the pain of the raw eczema that was still stinging and prickling over my arms, chest, and legs. I breathed deeply and took a stroll along the path near where I lived overlooking the sea. With wonder, my eyes began to take in exquisite patterns of light dancing through the trees, glittering rays of sunshine flickering on the hoods of cars, and the bright blue expanse of the sky. My ears attended to the music of the birds, the traffic, and the ocean in what seemed like meticulous detail. My spirit had come back to life. It became apparent that the deep assumption that there is something wrong with this moment was actually the very force that was making it *feel* wrong. Surrendering out of that, life flooded back to greet me with a mysterious benevolence and grace. It was as if a deeper intelligence in the universe was saying, "Yes, that's it my friend. That's what's always the case."

THE "PROBLEM"

Clearly not all experiences of bringing compassionate presence to our experience of physical pain will be that dramatic. Sometimes it may only feel like a tiny shift, especially in the beginning. However, this way of simplifying our relationship to unpleasant bodily sensations bears great fruit over time. It also begins to inform how we relate to all of life. The essence of the practice can be seen in the example above.

Connect to the sensations that are here with spaciousness and compassion. Feel underneath the mind's stories and the meaning it projects about the pain that is here. Hold those emotions and raw energies in your judgment-free awareness. Trust in the possibility of a radical freedom of heart right in this moment.

Whenever you reach the last step, there is a deep force you will inevitably meet—that which is saying "This is a problem." On the existential level, that assumption generates and solidifies the sense of suffering and anguish in the present moment. Meeting it directly and questioning its reality is powerful practice.

All of the negative stories that arise in the face of physical pain and discomfort have this one core assumption in common. If you reflect on the future scenarios that being in physical pain can spawn, such as "I can't go on feeling this way," stories about the past such as "It's been here so long," or perceptions of self in the present such as "I should have gotten rid of this by now. It's my fault," you'll observe that they all carry that core sense that this experience, right now, is a problem. It is wrong. It shouldn't be this way. Can you get a sense of this for yourself? This feeling often arises at the same time as the painful sensation itself. However, it is possible to begin to notice that they are actually separate phenomena. The early Buddhist texts differentiate these in a neat way. Pain or unpleasant bodily feeling is called *dukkha vedana*—pain on the level of sensation. The feeling of the problem, the wrongness or the existential dis-ease that accompanies it, is just called *dukkha*—suffering. Bodily pain has its own causes. Pain of being has its own as well. But they are not the same thing. Of course they can and do influence each other when our attention is caught in the storytelling mind, but ultimately they are two different dimensions of human experience. To realize this is liberating.

So what is painful sensation, anyway? When we attend to pain from the simplicity of awareness, what we find is an ever-changing field of sense impressions. What the conceptual mind thinks of as a fixed object in reality turns out to be far more amorphous and changeable. When we see and feel pain in the light of pure awareness, what we find is not as solid as we thought. It moves, ripples, disappears, and then returns. It isn't a fixed "thing." It is a series of events in a constant state of transformation. Seeing physical pain in this way can help us dislodge attention from the fixed perceptions that reinforce the sense of its stuck-ness and solidity.

In this process, we can also inquire into the painfulness of pain. What is it that makes pain painful? There is no answer to this question, by the way—it is an invitation to open the mind to a new way of seeing and inquiring. When we use this line of inquiry in an embodied, compassionate way, we often meet the other kind of pain at the same time—the pain of the heart, of our being, or of our reactions and emotional response to the presence of the sensations. We can then shift our attention to that feeling itself. What is it? Is it the same as the pain, or is it arising independently? Can it be softened? What thoughts keep it in place? What ways of looking at the present moment allow it to relax and recede? What shift of perspective is possible? This kind of inquiry opens up huge doors of possibility in the midst of our experience, just as it is.

REFUGE IN THE KNOWINGNESS

Investigating these two kinds of pain for ourselves is really the heart of finding freedom when our bodily experience is unpleasant and abrasive. It allows us to rediscover the freshness and aliveness of awareness itself, right in the midst of shut-down energy levels and painful sensations. Through unfolding the layers of perception and belief about what the pain means and connecting to the core emotions and gut feelings that are arising in response to physical pain, we are in the position to turn attention around and fall back into the richness of here-and-now presence. Releasing and relaxing the impulse to feed off unpleasant sensations in a way that amplifies our existential pain or dis-ease, our attention becomes steady enough to focus instead on our real home ground in the moment. This provides us with a crucial anchor when there is no way of relieving the physical sensations. It involves a shift of being and a trust that it is OK not to make the painful sensations our primary focus. Having quieted the stories and connected with the heart essence of our suffering in the moment, we can fall back into presence in this way. I have found this to be a source of real nourishment when there is no option for well-being on the physical level.

Abiding in the knowingness of mind is a direct practice. It cannot be explained or understood rationally. It is what happens when the open heart rests in itself rather than focusing on any object in particular. It is the silent but vital ground of every

175

moment underneath all the fabrications and time-bound narratives based around and spawning the person we take ourselves to be. On account of this, it is the ultimate simplicity, which we taste in the heart when we allow ourselves to be that simple too. Although being simple in the face of physical pain or discomfort is not often our first strategy, when the going gets tough, it is the very medicine that allows us to unhook from the suffering we have unconsciously been gnawing on. When we are simple, nothing needs to be made out of anything. To really feel this is a great joy. We have been let off the hook.

An inspiring lesson I received in the possibility of simplicity was from one of my main teachers in California, Ajahn Pasanno. Being the co-abbot of a training monastery, Ajahn Pasanno spent most of his time giving huge amounts of energy and attention to others. I was and continue to be in awe of his capacity for round-the-clock generosity and selfless giving. Living with him was a daily experience of being blown away. To this day I can't fathom how he did it. Long afternoons of receiving guests, followed by talking to the community at teatime, then offering teachings, and then sometimes sitting all night. If I had given a sixteenth of what he gave, I would have needed to spend a month in bed! So when it came time for Ajahn to have his annual period of self-retreat, it was understood that this was a very precious time. We were all delighted for him when the time came round for his quiet time in the forest in the Californian summer. It was after one of his solo retreats that I received a powerful lesson in the freedom that is possible in the midst of pain and discomfort. Instead of a blissful time of peaceful meditation in the forest, it turned out that Ajahn Pasanno's precious annual retreat had consisted of a barrage of intense gastrointestinal troubles. Hearing this, I was saddened. "Damn," I thought, "he must be so annoyed."

However, in the evening after he emerged from silence, he

came to sit right beside me as I was lounging on a cane chair in the warm evening. "Uh-oh, what have I done wrong?" was my initial thought. My teacher began to speak. "It's amazing," he said with a wonder and enthusiasm in his eyes that I wasn't expecting. "Huh?" I thought, caught quite off guard. "There was just the knowing. There was just awareness. In the middle of all that—the cramps, the stomach pain—I looked, and there was only the knowingness. That's all that was happening." I was taken aback. I hadn't expected that. In fact, I couldn't imagine it. But hearing it from my teacher in such a palpable and heartfelt way left an indelible impression on my consciousness. Perhaps because Ajahn Pasanno knew of the challenges I was facing, he thought to invite me into that possibility too. Indeed, at that point in time the condition of the body was a real struggle for me. To hear that another person could experience similar levels of pain and discomfort on the physical level and rest wholeheartedly in awareness itself was like a glimpse into a different universe—one that I deeply longed to inhabit. Those five minutes continue to be a source of light and inspiration for me in times of physical challenge and pain. I recall the steadfast clarity and openness that Ajahn Pasanno transmitted through his presence right in the middle of awful conditions and remember that it is possible to deeply let go. Because, when it comes down to it, why not?

MEDITATION ON BEING WITH PAIN

When we experience pain in the body, to begin with, it is important to establish an attitude of wisdom that will be sustainable.

The first thing to remember is that we're not trying to get rid of pain. This isn't an attempt to destroy, get rid of, or cut pain out of existence. Although this may be challenging, particularly if the experience of pain is intense, there is a great wisdom in this approach. When we enter into the practice with an open heart, we taste for ourselves how it actually works.

That in the mind that is setting pain up as an enemy and seeks to push it away actually increases the sense of pain being painful. It generates the sense that pain is unacceptable and can't be included in awareness. In contrast, what we are trying to feel into is an awareness that can be inclusive, sensitive, and awake, without holding to a sense that pain is "wrong." Through this the quality of pain begins to be felt as more amorphous, mysterious, and less stuck.

As we have seen already, the first step is to look at the relationship we have to pain in this very moment. So take a moment now to notice what perceptions, mind states, or attitudes are arising in relation to the felt experience of painful sensation. Shine the light of your curious awareness into this aspect of your inner experience.

It could be a sense of "I wish this would go away." Or maybe it's an underlying current of irritation and anger, such as "I hate this." Sometimes what we find is fear riffing on particular constructs of the future in the mind's eye. Try to taste these flavors of heart energy with no judgment. Trust in a radical, stripped-down awareness, free from commenting, measuring, or judging these states as "spiritual" or "unspiritual." Instead, just feel the whole sense of what is arising in this moment. Give yourself a few moments to do that right now.

Now see if you can expand awareness to touch the pain as well as the mind state. Notice that the mind state—the energy of heart and emotion—is not the pain. The pain itself is just so. The fear, anger, worry, or dislike is something that the heart is doing in this moment. We may not be doing it consciously—we may also be experiencing the results of habitual intentionality from the past—but it is something that can be either amplified or relaxed through choices we make in the present moment.

Allow attention to gently come into the hub of this activity of mind with a steady, open presence. Feel how it moves and flows. Inquire for yourself with the question "What function does this serve?" Ask this without harshness or judgment. It is an invitation for you to inquire directly into the mind state from a place of innocent inquiry. Don't assume anything. This is the only way intuitive wisdom can arise. Put the book down now, and spend a few moments with this inquiry.

Now shifting your attention slightly, see if you can get a sense of how that mind state affects the way the pain is received in awareness. You can even consciously amplify the thoughts of anger or fear to really sense what they do to the experience of painful sensation. Can you notice how they heighten the intensity of pain; how they make it seem like it is the whole of our conscious experience? They focus on it, amplify it, and make it seem huge.

In contrast, feel what it is like to trust that in yourself which can relax that contracted mind state, even to some degree. Relax the scenarios in the mind, the edges of tightness, and come back into a really simple presence. Return to a place of not-knowing in yourself. Sense into the possibility of being available to the very experience of the body right now. Feel into an open, receptive, porous awareness that includes the feelings of discomfort or pain that are here.

The trick with this approach is not to try to bring about a particular outcome but rather to relate to the mind and body in an experimental way. Notice what causes what in the present moment. It is like a science experiment in the context of the open, loving heart.

However, the general principle is that the simpler, the more open, the more innocent we can be with the experience of discomfort or pain, the more the sensations themselves can flow through awareness. They are allowed to be themselves. In doing this there is often an experience of discharging or releasing around the psychological pain that often accompanies them.

Attending in this way, a quality of compassion may begin to emerge. In the presence of physical pain, this can be felt as a silent but pervasive quality of heart. Can you feel that sense in yourself right now? It is compassion for the very pain of having a body that hurts. What is it like to fully feel the unpleasant and get that sense of "Yeah. This hurts"? Allow yourself to meet that hurting with the energy of compassion. Allow that compassion to suffuse your whole sense of yourself as you attend to it in this way. Take some time now to explore this possibility.

Compassion is a deeper quality than self-blame, hatred, or fear. It is the connection to what is most deeply human in the heart—your unobstructed human sensitivity. Allow this heart feeling of compassion to flow through the bodily system. Imagine it drenching the cells—up from the feet and circling through all the areas of the body as it is sensed in your awareness right now. Allow the whole sense of your body to be pervaded with this tender feeling of caring. Give yourself full permission to hold the difficult, the broken, in this vulnerable way. You can let yourself relax all the agendas, doubts, and inner violence. Be here in your own quiet, compassionate presence. This is great work you are doing. Trust that.

Through this process, the physical pain may not go away, but you have the opportunity to feel into a sense of freedom. While you may not be free of the sensations, can you feel the possibility of relaxing out of the core sense of affliction around the physical experience? Take a moment to seed awareness with this possibility.

What is it like to attune to freedom of heart in this moment? Can you sense the cooling, refreshing quality that comes about when your awareness is focused on this deep longing for release rather than caught in contracted judgments or reactions about the pain that is here? This freedom of heart isn't the freedom to control or to always make life as we want it, however. It is the here-and-now release from the sense that this moment is "wrong." Trust in an innocent, open kind of attention as you sit or lie here. Soften the edges of inner division. There is no need to divide yourself from yourself.

Keep inclining toward a relaxation on the cellular level. You can keep finding a refuge in nonreactivity and noncomplication. Allow awareness to encompass the body with as little need to fix, understand, or make a story out of it as possible. Expand and soften your attention so that it becomes a resonant field of knowing. Incline your heart toward relaxation and ease.

9

Unconditional Value

WHEN THE HEART is truly open and the mind is free from confusion, we recognize that all beings, including ourselves, are already valuable beyond comprehension. Nothing can quantify this value; nothing can be added to or subtracted from it. There is no distinction. This realization is radically different from how most cultures and societies think. As a species we are addicted to differentiation, judgment, and hierarchies of value. Our human mind seems to be wired to become entranced in this illusion. However, when we look and feel underneath the apparent reality of these fragmented perceptions of ourselves and others, we are struck by a whole new possibility. We begin to sense for ourselves that our ultimate value is never found through being somebody, achieving something, or proving anything. It is always right here and now in the sacredness and simplicity of being. It is not "mine" or "yours." It is the heart of experience itself.

Of course, on the social level distinctions do exist. Some people have greater skill and talent at some things than others. So, seen through a certain lens, these hierarchies have a relative truth: some people can run faster, sing better, or make more money than others. This is just the way of things. To taste our own unconditional value we don't need to deny the relative truth of this. What we do need to become clear about, however, is that these relative measurements, comparisons, and levels of skill never define our essential value. All of us will at some time lose these capacities. Old age, sickness, and death are the great levelers. When you live with chronic illness, pain, or disability, you will have already lost capacities you once had. Some of you will have lost a lot. Instead of causing you to live in a sense of lack, these losses can be turned around to take awareness to the taste of unconditional value in the heart of the present moment. There are wonderful treasures waiting there.

ALREADY HOME

When it comes to really connecting with and trusting our own unconditional value, the ability to rest in the sense of being at home in our ourselves, right here and now, is essential. On the level of conditions, things can get so bleak and trying when we are ill. There are times when there just isn't enough mental energy available to look the part, get things done, or be the person we feel we should be. Sometimes the mind just needs to rest. The place of true rest begins to reveal itself as a radical heart trust in our inherent OK-ness. When we give up solving anything or even needing to understand anything about the mind, the body's condition, or the future, we can then take that rest deeper into the nature of the present moment itself. Focusing on the ground of being right now is the doorway.

From one perspective, we are already home. We never left. Our true presence has always been here and now. It was never some other place or some other time. In order to truly taste this for ourselves, though, we need to be wise to when and how we feel we are *not* home, as we have already been doing in this book. Having become adept at this through a curious and non-judgmental inquiry into our own unique heart and mind, we can then move to a deeper level of inquiry: focusing on that quality of pure presence, or pure being itself, so as to bring it alive in this moment. While it is not a "thing" that can be grasped and in fact is always here and now regardless of the conditions of mind and sensations of body, there is a vital spark of awareness beneath the apparent reality of things that we can consciously attune to and begin to rest in *as* our own nature. Consciously connecting to awareness in this way involves the recognition that it is our real home ground and a trust in that reality, as we will see. When we become familiar with this paradigm shift, we can begin to abide in the feeling of our own unconditional value rather than continually selling it out to judgments and once-removed ideas of who we are or what others want us to be. This enables awareness to be experienced as an underlying ground that includes all states of mind—low or high, dark or bright. It is important to note here that while the concept of already being home itself offers some refreshment, holding on to a conceptual framework doesn't free the heart. There is a process involved. It is one that we can only travel ourselves through directly inquiring into the nature of presence in this very moment.

Inquiring into the quality of pure awareness itself has been a very powerful practice for me personally, as it connects to that dimension of ourselves that is always here, even when crashed out on the floor or completely exhausted. This kind of inquiry takes the knowingness or awareness at the heart of all experience as the primary object of meditation and contemplative inquiry. The beauty of this is that it doesn't depend on feeling great or even having a certain amount of mental energy. It isn't about manipulating conditions. Some of the most profound experiences of this kind of meditation have come for me on days when I have had to give up doing anything and instead just lie down in bed. The act of surrendering the outwardly seeking mind is itself a powerful foundation for peace. Rather than lying there feeling like a failure, however, we can take our inquiry deep into the fabric of the present moment. We can use our curiosity to see and feel underneath all the apparent definitions of "me" as a fixed thing in our mind's eye and instead connect intimately to that light of presence that is behind all mental imagery but always home. This kind of practice is the heart of many schools of Buddhism that have arisen throughout the ages. While my own personal training in this was in the Thai Forest tradition, where there is great emphasis on "being the knowing" and attending to "the one who knows," there are examples of this very same practice in Chinese and Japanese schools of Zen and Tibetan meditation schools. One can also find it in contemplative Christian practices such as centering prayer as taught by the wonderful Trappist monk Father Thomas Keating. Ultimately it points to the mind being aware of itself, or if you like, the heart resting in its own nature. In that way it is a universally human phenomenon and always takes us beyond words and ideas. When we attend to awareness we are already seeing through the limits of the conceptual mind and into the fabric of the present moment itself. So whatever words you yourself find useful as a conceptual framework are absolutely fine—these frameworks can only point our awareness to itself. They are, as they say in Zen, "The finger pointing at the moon," and not the moon itself. Please keep this in mind as I use words to describe the process below.

The heart of the inquiry is to notice the difference between all the objects of awareness, such as mental images, our inner voice, the sounds we are hearing, and the feelings in the body, and that which is *aware* of all of that. While the content of conditions is continually changing, there is something else, right here and now, that isn't changing. It is like space. It is like the light that makes it possible to see anything at all. What is that in yourself right now? Let this question saturate your experience of the moment. If the mind co-opts it with cynicism, gets lost in doubt, or tries to figure it out as a concept, then stop. Start again. Be innocent. Be fresh with each moment. What is awareness right now? Be aware of that. *Feel* that. *Be* that.

There is something ineffable about that, isn't there? You can't describe it, pin it down, or even define it. But it is always here. Do you notice how it comes more alive the more you focus on it? Can you feel the effects of this enlivening anywhere in your body, such as the center of your chest, your forehead, or all through your arms and legs perhaps? The process flows best when it is a continual plunging, a continual process of arriving fresh in the present moment and then letting go into this silent ground once again. Through this process we begin to feel our location shift from being caught in the fragmentation of mind, ideas, and sense impressions, back home into an undivided sense of presence. When we flip attention around to become aware of that which is aware, something comes alive in us. This feeling of aliveness comes right from the heart of ourselves and offers us a taste our own intrinsic value. It is similar to when you go outside and feel the sun on your face. You can't describe why, but you know it is valuable beyond measure. It makes life on earth possible. Plunging into awareness itself with all our heart and all our attention has a similar feeling. It restores us back to our own worth—not through creating an image with which to compare ourselves against others but by animating that sacredness of being that is our very nature and the nature of all those we share this planet with.

In this way, the practice of attending to awareness itself as the focus of our meditation has two effects: it allows us to see through the apparent reality of any state that is arising and also brings to life a heart-feeling of unconditional value. We feel at peace with ourselves, just as we are. It takes us out of the dream and into the real. Even if you taste the profound completeness of pure presence only once, you will never forget it. That taste ignites a longing that won't leave you. You will long to return home. You will also have a new context in which to relate to *all* ideas of who you are, as a this or a that. Those ideas, which often append themselves to the condition of the body, such as "I'm sick," are now seen in a different light. The body itself arises in the field of this awareness, so how could it ever define you? Awareness doesn't need to be healed, fixed, solved, or resolved. It is always in pristine condition.

Stories, on the other hand, are always looking for a resolution. They are always heading somewhere, fueled by the illusion of lack. We seek to resolve the "problem" with us by thinking more about ourselves. Something in us is unconsciously convinced, "If I just figure out what the problem with me is, then I'll be fine." This is the mind's primary tactic. When this seeking becomes infused with old habits of contracted and turbulent energy, it can be hard to find a way out. The first step is always to remember that none of that defines you. The second is to stop and feel how your wheels are spinning. Recognize that you are seeking something that isn't here. The last step is this coming back home to see and feel the context in which the seeking is taking place. We can switch our attention from trying to resolve the apparently never-ending wrongness with ourselves, our illness, or our life to the question "What is aware of all this, in this moment?" When we ask that question with sincerity and a heartfelt longing, it helps to dissolve the "world" and the "me" spawned by the problem-addicted mind. It allows us to come back home.

Placing attention on awareness with a contemplative interest in the nature of *right now* also takes a kind of innocent inquisitiveness. It isn't about generating more ideas and concepts, nor is it an effort to make ourselves into anything at all. It invites us into a recognition of the timeless dimension of ourselves. We begin to recognize that there is something about who and what we are in this moment that has always been here. We can never put our finger on it or even grasp it with our rational mind, but when we look, we see. There is this awake aliveness that was always here, behind the five-year-old we once were, the teen-ager, and the adult we are now. Think back to all the people you have felt yourself to be in your life. How many people have you been? It can be amazing to remember how it felt to be five years old, for example, and at the same time remember that which *knew* that person you felt yourself to be. What is that? Fall back into that for a moment without trying to figure anything out about it at all. Can you sense the timelessness of that? Whatever that something is, it isn't traveling anywhere in time, nor has it been anywhere. Isn't that amazing?

It is the same on a day-to-day level also. Think again about all the people you have felt yourself to be today. This is subtle and takes a refined kind of remembering, but see if you can get a sense of that. Who did you feel yourself to be when you woke up? How did the sense of that person change as you had break-fast or your morning drink? How has it been evolving over the course of the day? How many different "people" have you felt yourself to be in the last half hour? Now bring the fact of their impermanence into your heart. They all changed, didn't they? None of them stuck around forever. Tasting for yourself that all these images and identities come and go, arise and cease, opens up a sense of perspective in the heart and mind. It allows you to focus directly on the timeless dimension of yourself, which is where true, unconditional value always lies waiting. This recog-nition invites you to rest in the energy of awareness as your real ground. The more you allow yourself to let go into this ground, the more skilled you will become at staying connected to it throughout your daily life, your relationships, and your responsibilities.

THE SWORD OF WISDOM

Sometimes, however, this kind of inquiry will not be enough. The energy of the ego-mind can be tenacious. When the only conditions it can rummage through to find a definition of meaning or worth are the pain, losses, and apparent failures involved in living with illness, it can embed itself in our awareness as a background of depression, heaviness, or dejection. When left unattended, it wreaks havoc on our emotional and mental well-being. When nothing else will shift it, you need a sword.

In contemplative traditions, the metaphor of the "sword of wisdom" is one that has been used throughout the ages. It refers to that strength of mind, of awareness that can slice through the wall of fabricated sludge dragging us into suffering. It is that which says "I know what you are. I'm not buying it." Although it is clear and strong, it is not violence. It is what violence wants to be but fails at. It is liberating wisdom. When the mind is submerged in a maze of depressive, perhaps conflicting identities, or weighed down by the apparent reality of "Who I have become," the sword is needed. When kindness, patience, and even insight just don't seem to have any effect, it is often an indicator that new energy is required in the present moment. You can't force it, however—there is a right time for it, and only you will know when that is. Trying to slice a mind state to bits never works and can easily lead to dissociative states, as we have seen. The sword of wisdom is more subtle than that—it is the heart responding to the call to wake up. It is what happens when we see the misery the mind is pulling us down into, and our spirit rises up with an audacious "No!" It is a liberating force in the heart. I have been

190

surprised by it on many occasions—often when things appeared most hopeless and stuck. At the heart of it has always been a sudden waking up out of ideas and feelings based on what illness means about me and my ultimate value.

One of the first times I was shown the power of this sword-like quality of awareness was in dialogue with my teacher Ajahn Amaro during my time in Northern California. After many years of living within the monk's life in the context of debilitating illness, my mind had become obsessed with images and views of what a "real monk" looked like and was bombarding itself with judgments in relation to these ideals. Many daily experiences of not being able to *look* the part, such as frequently leaning forward on my face in meditation, eating special food, and not being able to take part in manual work in the forest with the community, played into the bias of identifying with those forms as being absolute definitions of value. If I couldn't live up to them, I was a useless monk, I thought. This identification gave rise to a whirling undercurrent of doubt. Though part of me knew this was all made up, the energy of doubt was strong. I would try to counter it by saying "But I *am* good. I *am* worthy. I *do* belong here," and yet the force of doubt would pull awareness down into its hole. "Do I? I mean, look at all these things I'm failing at. I'm worthless." Underpinning this entire maze of thoughts was the core assumption that my ultimate value could be found in an image of "me" based on what I can or can't do. As long as awareness remained directed outward into this realm of ideation and fabrication, it felt bound to the paradigm of measurements, comparisons, up and down, better and worse. Gradually the effect of this constant turmoil took its toll, and it felt easier to resign to the thought "I give up. I'm out of here." There was a kind of peace in that: I knew I was a failure and I could just accept it and leave. With this newfound resolve in mind, I strode out of my hut in the middle of the afternoon on a mission to find Ajahn Amaro, who I knew was down in his office at the time. I was going to tell him I'd realized I was a fraud and I was leaving. Simple. Clean. "Let's do this," I thought.

Exhausted and hungry, as was often the case, I knocked on Ajahn Amaro's office door and slunk meekly into a seat. "How can I help you?" he asked, smiling warmly. "Well," I began, "I've been thinking. You know . . . I've realized I don't belong here. I'm not a good *bhikkhu* [monk]. There's just so much I can't do. I'm a burden on the community. I've realized that I should just leave." It felt scary to say this out loud, and my body flushed with fear upon revealing these hitherto unexpressed perceptions of myself. He listened, unfazed, and looked clearly into my eyes for some time. I prepared myself for a response such as, "Oh, I'm sorry you feel that way; let's talk it through," as had often been his compassionate and patient approach in the years leading up to this moment. What I got was something quite different.

"It's self-view," Ajahn Amaro said, clearly and firmly in his English schoolteacher accent. "Huh?" I asked. "That's just self-view. It's delusion," he continued. "It's not who you are. Let it go."

His unwavering presence was both frightening and deeply compelling. I stared back at him and felt the power of that clarity. There was a long silence. The same sword that he had manifested in his response arose in my own being. I felt it cutting through the swamp of my self-obsessed convictions.

"*Whoa*," I replied. There was more silence, but now with the addition of huge grins. "Can I really trust that?" I asked. "Is it that simple?" "Yes," replied my teacher.

Ajahn Amaro showed me something profound that day. The power and clarity of his presence lay in his refusal to even entertain the stories I was presenting as real. As a result, I was offered a taste of that very possibility for myself. I liked it. Although it felt new and fresh and wobbly, it also felt like falling back into a dimension of clarity that had been hidden. Wisdom was the key.

Self-view was the lock. This meeting sparked a hunger in me—one that longed to really understand how the habit of undermining my own value worked and what I could do to unhook it from awareness. The Buddha's teaching on the first three fetters of mind, to which Ajahn Amaro was referring that day, became the perfect framework for seeing through the maze of dejected thoughts I was being assailed with.

USING THE SWORD

These "fetters," or shackles of mind, refer to the tendency of *selfing* as it arises, moves, and gets stuck in our awareness. Selfing is the activity of mind that looks to find a real self through imagining a world "out there" that is judging and measuring "me," or the sense of "me in time," which looks to find itself though questions like "Who am I now compared to who I was when I was healthy?" or "Where am I now compared to where I could have been at this stage of my life?" It refers to whenever the mind feeds upon an image of oneself as being absolutely true and becomes identified with the emotions that arise in relation to that image. For example, on a day when I am lying on the couch exhausted, unable to even reply to e-mails, I notice this force stirring in the belly and looking for an object in the mind. It can arise as the sense of time in the form of "You were so much better last year. It's all going downhill," or the sense of a "them" muttering in the peripheries of the mind, "Oh, dear. Not very useful today, are you?" This tendency relates intimately to the drives of *becoming* we explored earlier in the context of allowing deep rest. This very primal habit of getting stuck in selfing is the root of all the ways we undermine our own connection to unconditional value in the present moment.

Selfing is a subtle kind of closing that obscures the ease and peace of resting in awareness we've been exploring in this chapter. When it is not seen for what it is, it easily drags us down and limits both our happiness and our capacity for loving fully. Understanding these fetters of mind is always a process of dropping away. The journey into freedom is not a process of acquisition but a gradual letting go and releasing from these forms of mental imprisonment. I find this perspective very optimistic, especially given the limitations that come through living with diminished energy levels and power of control. It is wonderful to think of the process of freedom and awakening as one of unfolding into what is already true, right here, rather than a struggle to manipulate conditions or our sense of self into some far-off ideal. Coming to know the first three of these fetters of mind activates a paradigm shift that undoes the tenacious feelings of diminished value that often accompany our sense of who we are when the body is ill and incapacitated. It opens us up to a simplicity of being so natural and uncontrived that the self-seeking mind can miss it for a lifetime.

This first of these fetters is self-view. We know it anytime our attention is stuck on an image of ourselves, frozen in time, believing it is who we really are. Seeing through self-view doesn't mean we will not or should not have an everyday sense of self or be able to refer to ourselves as a person. That is normal and necessary and part of being human. Our self-sense matures with wisdom and brightens with kindness and compassion. It is a necessary basis for finding meaning and value in our lives and for living in a way that we truly respect. Self-view is when it becomes a mask we are looking at, measuring, and taking to be permanently "me." Even though some of these masks may have been hanging around the peripheries of awareness for a very long time, they all share one thing in common: they are stuff the mind made up. They're fake. Through aligning the sword of wisdom to our deep desire for freedom of heart, we begin to see for ourselves that none of these images are actually who we are.

How could we see them if they actually were us? How could they keep changing if they were a real identity? If you think back to the last ten minutes or the last hour, can you notice how the views, perceptions, or assessments that you have of yourself have been changing, morphing, blooming into being, and then transforming into something else again? When they are present in the mind, we feel that they are permanent and that we have always been them. As soon as we open up some space in the mind, we begin to see that this is not the case. It is a trick. We can learn to see through it.

Coming to know the myriad ways our mind and heart gets caught in the masks of self-view also involves a radical kind of trust in the heart. This trust allows us to resist the force of the second fetter that often lurks as an energetic experience underneath the view of ourselves we believe is real: *doubt*. This doubt is the energetic component of selfing. It is that which is seeking to define ourselves as either a this or a that. It asks questions based on the premise that we can find ourselves through thought, images, or ideas. "Am I good?" "Am I bad?" "Am I deserving?" "Am I likable?" are questions that doubt conjures into being—often in subterranean, insidious ways we don't see. There is something in the human mind that is convinced that there will be some kind of answer to these questions, so it conceives of self-views in order to try to satisfy the energy of doubt. However, when we can remain grounded in the embodied experience of the present moment, we can begin to unhook from these strategies of allaying doubt and actually contact it as an energetic movement in the belly or the chest. We can then *feel* what it is. It is an uncomfortable kind of not-knowing that believes it can't rest until it knows for sure. What it doesn't see is that it is looking in the wrong place, in a way that reinforces (rather than allays) the discomfort. This doubt is the force that doesn't allow the mind to rest on one self-image as ever being true. One moment we think,

"Ah, I'm a good person. I'm great." The next moment someone says something unkind or offhand and we can begin to think, "Oh, wait, am I? Maybe I'm not. I knew it. Or did I?" This is doubt in action. This doubt is always connected to our sense of value. It doesn't refer to the practical, everyday kind of doubts that can be useful, such as the ability to remember our actions or speech and discern whether or not they were useful, or try to understand where they were coming from in ourselves. This is an important faculty that is of benefit to our well-being. What it refers to, in my experience, is doubt about whether or not we are fine as we are. Whether we have value. Although grasping the energy and seeking to reassure it through referring to positive images can of course have a practical function, this strategy remains vulnerable to change and is ultimately unstable. Understanding and unhooking from the energy of doubt itself is where freedom really lies.

Being with the energy of doubt without trying to satisfy it through an answer can be a challenging process, however. In my experience it takes repeated attempts and a willingness to fail, then try again, then fail once more. Because it is a such a counterintuitive way of relating to the present moment, you will need to train awareness to attend in this way. The key is to identify the flavor of doubt within a particular story that is playing out in the mind. It takes a stepping out of content, and a feeling-awareness of the underlying *taste* in the body and heart. When we see "Ah, this is doubt. It's just doubt," then we can begin to practice consciously letting it *be* doubt, but not trying to solve it. It sounds radical, and it is. But within that resolve and steadfastness, the energy of doubt begins to subside and release. Letting go of doubt doesn't mean finally having answered the question "Am I valuable?" It comes through letting the question burn, writhe, and flail in heart presence until the energy runs out. With the perspective that no image can ever define you, it is possible to create the space for this transformation. It may feel weird or somehow naughty and irresponsible—but don't give in to those thoughts. By not grabbing hold of doubt, the heart is actually affirming its own unconditional value at the same time. It is the recognition that what we really are is already whole, already valuable beyond measure. It is the process of not selling out that value.

The third of these fetters of mind is a habit in the heart and mind that can be translated as *clinging to conventions.* The Pali phrase is *silabata paramasa,* which literally means "fondling ways of behaving." It is a significant force to come to know in ourselves, because it is one of the main ways that the mind's selfing tendency coagulates into a barrier to freedom of heart. While the historical Buddha never recommended clinging to a view that all conventions should be discarded (which is another place that our self-view can try to hang out), what he did encourage was a wisdom regarding how we identify with them as being absolutely real. When our bodies are ill, there are many subtle ways that the mind can get caught in this belief around the "right" way of doing things and judge ourselves because we are no longer a person who can do them. The mind projects an ideal self that we should be, just *over there,* splits off from it, and feels that if only we were that person, then we would have value. An everyday example that I have hit against in myself time and time again is around "being useful." We should all be useful, right? Surely being "spiritual" means saving the world, right? That's what my mind can believe, anyway. This becomes a problem on days when there is hardly enough energy to go into the kitchen to make a cup of tea—let alone leave the house to do wonderful things for countless beings. Of course, helping others and doing good is a wonderful thing, and when there is energy, I always love it. But when I have no choice but to surrender the whole day or week for rest and healing, then I feel the rub of my clinging. The inability to live up to a conventional image of the "good me" then becomes a burden lingering in the peripheries of the mind and weighing on the heart when I need rest. If this isn't seen, it can easily turn into a externalized version of the self-view: a "them" out there tut-tutting because I haven't lived up to society's expectations of being the right kind of person. "I haven't been useful, and therefore I am not worthy," goes the refrain. Yet all of this is unnecessary. Appending my value to an idea of fitting into conventions—even spiritual or functional ones—always ends up in a heart needlessly suffering.

There are other, more subtle ways this tendency operates as well. Some of the ones I encounter in myself are ideas like "Spiritual people are always happy, and definitely not fed up and grumpy like I am today," "A *real* practitioner would spend all night burning in the fire of their pain instead watching a movie like I am," and the old favorite, "If I were practicing meditation right, my body wouldn't be ill." Do these sound familiar? The key is to become interested in how you, yourself, get stuck in the belief that how well or how "normally" you can do something is what *defines* you, and therefore defines your absolute value. Seeing through this tendency to measure worth against how well we can fit in to a convention of "doing it right" is a powerful skill to cultivate. It directly looks at where we assume and perpetuate an inherent lack of value and freedom. At the heart of things, conventions never define us. They can be useful and beneficial to ourselves and others on the relative level, but ultimately all of these human-made forms and expectations are there to be related to, not identified with. When we identify with them, we suffer.

Looking at the first three fetters of mind in this way is what is often called the *via negativa* of contemplative practice. It is a process of deconstruction. With these three general areas of selfing as a template, we can gradually become wise to our own habits of mistaken identity and begin to peel away the layers of apparent reality they squeeze the mind and heart into. In doing this we unpack, unbind, and release our awareness from the fabrications it is habituated to believe in as "me." This process involves a kind of clarity and resolve that takes time to cultivate. A loving and open heart is the prerequisite for this journey into the hub of selfing. If there isn't a warm, benevolent attitude at the heart of our inquiry, things can go very wonky. Indeed, in my experience, the fullness and warmth of heart that comes from nurturing the quality of kindness has been a necessary foundation for opening deeper out of the constructions of self-view. The energy underlying these shackles of mind can be very powerful, so it needs to be approached with sensitivity. A trap that I became caught in in my early years of committed practice was to try to obliterate self-view out of existence using willpower and force. Because this was coming from an inner harshness and an aversion to myself just as I was, the result was that the forces of doubt and self-criticism increased rather than decreased. The only difference was that now the object of self-view was the "me who should get rid of self-view but can't, so has failed because of that"! The mind can be a tricky place. As opposed to willful or even violent approaches to deconstructing the matrix of self-view, we can find an attitude of acceptance and openheartedness that is coupled with a strength and clarity of mind. Our strength and resolve is then in service of the well-being and embodied engagement that is already present rather than being co-opted by the spiritual ego that secretly wants to get away from our human heart and mind. This process of deconstruction is therefore a loving one. It is love saying, "Wow—this image I am taking to be 'me' is painful. It hurts. It limits me. I'm going to be strong in not giving in to it. I'm going to see it for what it is." In that way, the *via negativa* acts in service of the positive, the optimistic, and the whole rather than turning into the "path of negativity." Don't travel down that road.

FINDING VALUE IN EVERYDAY LIFE

Although we have been focusing on the capacity to access a core trust in our own unconditional value, it is important not to overlook the more everyday ways of connecting to value and meaning that are possible even in the midst of a life of illness or disability. In terms of our inner life, a commitment to compassion, generosity, and the open heart go a long way in terms of safeguarding and nourishing a sense of self-respect on a day-to-day level. From the perspective of causality in the realm of mental well-being, our actions and speech in everyday life matter. Because they matter, they have power. This power can either obstruct or support the connection to unconditional value in our hearts. If we don't attend to these, it is hard to let go deeper into the simplicity of unconditional value in presence itself. For example, if we live from a place of harshness, cruelty, or deceit, that will inevitably create a wall in the heart that solidifies tendencies toward guilt, self-blame, and other forces that suck the mind into a hole of apparent deficiency. This harshness can take place in the form of either the myriad internal ways of harming ourselves we have come to know in this book or the same energy directed toward others. In the process of direct inquiry that has been unfolding for you, you may have begun to encounter more subtle layers of unkind, dark, or murky intentions that infiltrate the way you relate to others. This is normal. It's just how it goes—for all of us. Rather than judging yourself for what you find, the way of wisdom is the way of curiosity. You can look at what drives you, what motivates you, and really get clear about what effects acting out these forces have in your own heart and mind. This is a personal inquiry. You have to taste it for yourself.

On the other hand, making a commitment to live from the open, wise heart generates a kind of self-respect that, while still dependent and conditioned upon things we "do," gives rise to a quiet feeling of satisfaction in ourselves. This satisfaction is deeper than just feeling good on the level of sensation. It can be present as a kind of warm contentment even while the body is weighed down by pain and discomfort. While this level of doing doesn't entail performing amazing feats and may not require much energy at all, it is still a meaningful kind of intentional action that gives our encounters with others meaning. As an old Forest Master once put it, it is like learning the "craft of the heart." Exploring this realm of the everyday, the seemingly mundane, we gradually learn how to align our actions and speech with our deepest aspiration for value. We begin to see how the two are entwined and realize how this process is actually always going on. The opportunity to align speech and action with kindness, goodness, and the undivided heart is there every moment. Putting our trust in this way of being can bring great gladness and meaning to a day when options for performing tasks, being someone, or even being conventionally "useful" have gone out the window.

In attending to our day-to-day intentions, however, it is essential not to cling to an idea of who we think we are according to whether or not we have performed according to some ideal or another. This very quickly becomes self-view and can easily trap the mind into a cul-de-sac of lack and feelings of not measuring up. It keeps the thinking mind spinning within the need to measure and assess ourselves. Memory can become tyrannical. I recall a period in my life where I began measuring myself against an imagined daily "quota" of generous actions in order to assess whether or not I was worthy of my own respect. I had totally missed the point! So, rather than using the aspiration to kindness and goodness as another way to beat ourselves up through focusing on all the ways we perceive we are getting it "wrong" (which is more of the same inner division), the point is to engage in our aspiration pragmatically and allow ourselves to explore the effects. When we are ill, there are many ways we will not be "perfect" according to an ideal. We will fail, forget, become lost in turbulence, sink into sludge, and then rise up again. Luckily, getting rid of this flow isn't the point. The real perfection comes through relaxing out of the whole need to rest upon an image of ourselves as good or bad, worthy or unworthy, in the midst of the ever-changing conditions of our physical and mental landscape. There is no substitute for that.

GUIDED MEDITATION ON UNCONDITIONAL VALUE

Find a posture that is restful, relaxed, and suitable for your condition right now. It may be sitting on a seat, lying down in a way that still allows you to be alert and bright, or in a meditation position on a cushion. Take some time to get comfortable.

In your direct, embodied awareness, attend to the flow of the breath as you feel it in the body. Return to the core sense of presence that is aware of that right now.

Relax the grip on the stories of the mind. Let them be there, but soften out of the need to give weight to whatever worlds or personae they are presenting in your mind's eye. Feel into the center of the chest and the pit of the belly—the energetic location of who you feel yourself to be. In this direct awareness, see if you can feel wherever there may be a "me" that is being clung to. Take a few moments to get a readout on what this moment is saying about that "me" you might be, shouldn't be, or once were.

Now relax around the story of "me" and place your attention upon the feeling of clinging itself. How does that feel? What is it like? Where can you feel it? With an all-encompassing awareness, feel the feeling of that clinging.

Sense your awareness moving around it, observing it as if from all angles—like a camera circling around and in and back again. See if you can apply the same spaciousness to the core images and ideas at the heart of that clinging. Relax the identification with that as being what you really are right now. Instead, be curious, open, aware. Explore this possibility for as long as you like.

Now see if you can also give your attention to the relaxed yet bright awareness that knows the very feeling of me and the mask it is presenting as "myself." Drop back into that feeling sense of presence. Underneath the worlds the self-view may be spawning, this awareness doesn't have a definition to it. It remains undefined yet fresh and alive. Can you sense that at the heart of your experience right now? That which is looking out is not a mask.

Soften into that field of looking, of pure sensing, which has no definition. While the mask may still be there as an image or a tight feeling in the chest, you can still fall back into the absolute simplicity underneath it. A vibrant, subtle awake-ness.

Trust that right now you don't have to be anything at all. You have full permission to just be here. That is more than enough. It is unfathomably enough. The perfection is right here and now unconditionally.

Feel that in your heart of hearts. Sense the expansiveness, the timelessness of that. It doesn't need anything added to it. Nothing can be taken away from it. It is neither yours nor mine—it just is, always. Fall back into that perfection.

10

Letting Go

THE HEART OF ALL the practices and perspectives offered in
this book is the capacity to let go. You may not have noticed it,
but you have been letting go a lot already. Every time you have
seen through a story the mind has taken to be real, released the
grip of self-judgment, or softened around anger and despair,
there is something you have had to let go of. The act of letting go
is what keeps us sane. If we couldn't let go of all the stuff that
floats to the surface of the mind, all the crazy thoughts and wayward intentions, we wouldn't even be able to survive a day with
illness and pain. So letting go is something we do all the time.
This skill has great transformative power when it is aligned with
wisdom and kindness. In the process of finding freedom of heart
and peace of mind within the experience of illness, it is always
an ally. You could use other words to describe this ability we
have. Sometimes it is felt as the act of surrender, as is the case
with true acceptance. Often it is the act of coming into the fullness of the present-moment experience in all its messy imperfec-
tion. When we are in pain or limited in energy, we know we

can't "go" anywhere else. We may not like it, but we know it is the case. So letting go means surrendering deeply to what is here right now—and out of the sense of the problem. At other times it is felt as a process of release—we feel as if we are releasing the grip on experience or the mind's clinging to a particular state, mood, or feeling. And when it comes to the heart, letting go is opening. It is the experience of widening, deepening, and softening that comes when we trust in the healing energy of kindness and generosity to ourselves; when we let it suffuse our sense of being alive.

THE FACT OF IMPERMANENCE

Letting go relies on a basic characteristic that all states of mind, experiences, and feelings share in common: impermanence. You will have already noticed this quality whenever you have brought awareness to the ever-changing content of your thinking mind or the deeper layer of masks and images of self-view at the heart of particular states. When the Buddha himself taught about the nature of experience, he was unequivocal about the significance and scope of impermanence. What is impermanent? All conditioned things. What are "conditioned things"? Rather than being things "out there," the teaching on impermanence directs us back home to our actual experience in any given moment. It is designed to free the heart from the suffering that comes when we cling to that which is always of the nature to change, dissolve, or die. It shows us how and where to let go. So the conditioned things spoken of in the ancient texts are those that can be experienced in our awareness right now: the body, feelings, ideas, states, and self-views. On a day-to-day level all of these facets of our present-moment experience are in a process of movement, transition, appearing, and disappearing. Some change slower than others, but they are all of the same nature. Have you ever noticed this? Take minute now to close your eyes and get a feeling for this. Resting in the soft strength of presence you have already been cultivating, feel what it is like to abide as the knowingness itself while everything in experience, seen, felt, or thought, is allowed to arise, present its case, and then fade out. Taste the letting go that comes with that shift.

Training the mind to recognize and trust in the fact of impermanence gradually forges a recognition in the core of our being. This recognition, which is heart-wisdom, is crucial when it comes to finding peace in the face of the many kinds of inevitable impermanence illness reveals to us through the loss of who we once were, what we could once achieve, what we once looked like, or how our body used to feel. In many ways illness is itself an endless teaching on impermanence. It shows us what is always the case for all beings on this planet. It often does so in stark and unwanted ways. In the face of these changes, do we know how to wisely let go? In my own experience letting go only became more than just a nice idea, or a mental posture, when I began to investigate what it really is that can be let go of anyway. Consciously investigating the impermanence of not just the macro level, but also the micro level—the components of mind and body that form an apparent reality that we mostly look *out of* but rarely look *at*—continues to be an essential part of this process.

When the Buddha talked about all "conditioned things" being impermanent, he often summed them up as five different categories of experience that we can see and feel for ourselves in any given moment. Taken as a whole they cover any kind of experience of conditions that we can have as human beings. Termed the five *khandas* in Pali, or *skandhas* in Sanksrit, these groups or "aggregates" of experience all interact with and feed off each other. I have found it very potent to explore these as present-moment phenomena, and the investigation into what those ancient texts were referring to has itself been a revelatory process. As with all different aspects of meditation and contemplative inquiry, direct exploration has been the key.

The first category of experience is the body—this realm of materiality itself. It refers to the "body-ness" of body—the fact that there is this material form here, right now. There are your hands holding this book, there are your feet touching the ground, there is this face of ours, these eyes, these organs in here somewhere, and the layer of skin covering it all. This is the vehicle for the other four *khandas*. We all know that the body is impermanent, don't we? Or do we? Conceptually we may think, "Yeah, yeah, of course the body is impermanent . . ." but how often do we actually take this fact in? Although we all know these bodies of ours are going to disappear one day, as food for worms or smoke floating up into the sky, not many of us in the West seem all that keen on exploring the implications of this. On the contrary, our culture idolizes the body as if it were the absolute measure of identity. As if it were permanence itself. It is a natural human tendency to do this. You don't have to look very far online before you are bombarded with ads telling you how to look great, lose fat, lose wrinkles, get an incredible tan or six-pack abs in four weeks, and so on. And yet if you are living with a body that is out of your personal control, that you wouldn't be able to squeeze into these tightly defined ideals of bodily form even if you tried, all of those messages become oppressive. Tuning in to the impermanence of the body, on the other hand, eases the mind out of that sense of oppression or obsession. It doesn't mean becoming morbid or in any way generating a negative view of the body. That is just the other extreme, and not the Middle Way, which remains our compass for wisdom and clear seeing. It is just about facing facts as they are, not as we think they should be. Aging happens, death happens. To everyone. The Buddha encouraged his students to contemplate skeletons and to then recognize that "one day, that will be this body here."

When done with calm and a real interest in waking up out of a negative bodily image or being fixated upon a particular physical manifestation of our illness that we don't like, this kind of contemplation is a soothing balm. We remember that we can let go. Directly perceiving the impermanence of the body in this way brings us face to face with the fact that holding on to the body, the way it looks or what it can do, is grabbing hold of that which ultimately will never be lasting. It will never provide an enduring refuge. In the middle of difficult times when my body is in pain or refusing to function, I find this recollection to be a welcome relief. It reminds me that this body here is not where perfection lies. So where is the real perfection? What is your real home right now?

Directly arising from this body of ours is the second of the *khandas*: sensory consciousness. The senses of tactile sensation, sight, sound, smell, and taste are the only way we can know anything. They make up everything that we consider to be "me, right here." For example, "My body feels this way" refers to tactile sensation, while "What I look like" refers to sight. It is fascinating to focus directly on each one of the senses anew in this way—with a sense of curiosity and wonder. What are these faculties anyway? What is seeing? What is listening? Focusing on the senses in a deliberate way from the position of awareness is an instant teaching in impermanence. Look at something, then close your eyes. Where did the image go? Notice sounds arising in your immediate environment, such as a car driving past or a bird chirping. They arise, then vanish, just like that. In Buddhist texts, there is a sixth sense that is added to these: thinking. Thinking is the sensory vehicle in which all of our worlds, identities, futures, and pasts are arising. Like the sound of a bird, it is always arising right now. All thoughts arise now. Every single one. All thoughts cease now. If we notice.

The third of the *khandas* is the category of feeling we have explored in chapter 8. Coming to know those three areas of pleasant, unpleasant, and neutral feeling opens us up to a more universal perspective on the experience of the senses. As we have seen, it takes us underneath and out of the particular story appended to what is happening right now and into the fundamental feeling tone of pleasure, displeasure, or neutrality in this moment. It allows us to widen the aperture of awareness to get the whole sense of how this moment feels and how that feeling is affecting us. This is how it helps us to let go. However, the quality of feeling also applies to the realm of mind—we not only sense these three types of feeling in relation to bodily sensation but also in terms of our heart-feeling in response to stimuli on the level of the senses, or thought itself. If we have a thought we would rather not have, it can suffuse the mind with unpleasant feeling. If someone says something harsh or unkind, we feel it in our guts. If someone says we are wonderful, we feel that too. If someone says, "I forgot to call so and so," we may feel a neutral feeling, a kind of "Oh, OK. That's a fact that I am registering now, but it doesn't affect me on a feeling level." Directly discerning the impermanence of this domain of mind is essential when it comes to letting go of negative or self-defeating mind states. It allows us to pan out and connect to the primary heart-tone that is giving rise to a perception about what our situation means. Whenever we take this level of mental feeling to be absolutely real, permanent, and true, we set ourselves up for suffering. When we cling tightly to a feeling of unpleasantness, such as the distaste or "yuck" that can arise in relation to our own body when it is ill, we take it to be permanent and true. "This sucks" and "I hate it" follow on in a flash. Yet the unpleasant feeling is not a fixed, permanent reality. It is a momentary response. When we release the grip of attention, we avail ourselves to the whole range of possibilities on the level of mental feeling. The light of awareness shines as a result.

Feeling is often said to go hand in hand with the fourth *khanda*: perception. The Pali word, *sanna,* literally means "sign," and refers specifically to the take we have on any given sense impression, thought, person, or event. It is that which shapes unpleasantness into "unacceptable" and pleasantness into "the best thing ever." It is the faculty that perceives another person to be "threatening," "my friend," "desirable," "a bit suspect," and so on. It scans experience and looks for definitions through which to interpret it. It often arises in a flash, accompanied by one of the three kinds of feeling. Awareness gets pulled into it and we then find ourselves looking *out* of it, and often forgetting that it is something that arose in the present moment. In this way perception is often like a pair of sunglasses we have forgotten we are wearing. It isn't actually our eyes. It is not an absolute reality. Of course the approximations and filters of meaning that perception provides us with are essential for living a human life. Many of them are neither here nor there—they are purely functional ways of navigating the world. Many of them provide us with comfort, the ability to appreciate beauty, to understand affection, and to delight in the presence of others. But underlying all of them is the fact of impermanence. None of them can be held on to or manipulated into being permanently present. They have their own life span. When it comes to the ones at the root of states of distress or suffering, the capacity to sense the impermanence of these subtle perceptions is an enormous blessing. It allows awareness to hone right in on the primary assumptions that are generating stress or anguish. Underneath the many kinds of self-view we explored in the previous chapter, for example, can be a very basic perception feeding off a feeling. In the example of my attempt to leave the monk's life, the perception I came to know was a simple one, but it was taken to be real, fixed, not open to questioning and absolute. It was the perception of "wrong." Once that was grasped, hold of it extended out onto everything it saw, thought of, and remembered about my life. And it didn't take long for it to weave a "me" poisoned with that same "wrongness" into being. It was all perception.

The fifth of these categories of experience is called *sankhara* in Pali. My favorite translation of this is "volitional formations." It refers to the fabricating tendency of mind—the ability to replicate, reproduce, and re-create worlds of self and other out of perception and feeling. These formations are volitional because they are moved and shaped by currents of impulse in the heart. If we attend underneath any story that is arising in the present moment, we can *feel* this volitional drive in the space of embodied presence. It is that which pushes away, hankers after, or holds on to. It is primarily moved by liking or not liking, wanting or not wanting. So *sankhara* is a very deep and subtle aspect of mind. It is that which moves us and that we are moved by. Exploring the impermanence of *sankhara* is at its heart an energy practice. It involves handling an energetic sense of the mind in the present moment with clear, grounded awareness. It is the skill you have already been cultivating in yourself through attending to the difference between self-harm and kindness in the heart, being present and open with turbulent energies of anger or fear, and exploring the way the heart closes into the sense of "the problem." *Sankhara* is the force underlying all of that. It is that which makes something out of anything. I find it useful to feel what this force is in the stillness and quietness of meditation. When the mind is settled and collected, I can feel the difference between awareness itself, which isn't moving or changing, and the energy of *sankhara,* which is always looking to make something, find something, understand something, or be someone. Stepping back out of where it tries to take awareness, I recognize that it too is of the nature to change. However, we don't have to get rid of it to see that it changes. It is more a mat-

ter of aligning ourselves with that which is immutably present—
being that presence itself. So we can let *sankhara* do its thing
however it wants, but we let go into non-movement. The seeking
goes on, but we stop looking for anything. This is a wonderful
possibility to explore in meditation.

If you are low on energy, you may find those five categories
a bit too much to focus on right now. That is totally fine. There
are days when I can investigate these in the quiet space of meditation or in the midst of the flow of everyday life, and there are
days when I can't. However, coming to know them, gradually
and directly, has opened me up to the true meaning of impermanence and continues to do so. Impermanence isn't a concept or a
belief. It is a fact. Witnessing it firsthand on all of these subtle
levels of present-moment experience allows us to wake up. What
initially seems like a hardened bundle of suffering is gradually
unfolded and softened through letting in the impermanence of
all the forces and assumptions that make it up. Letting in the
fact of impermanence is letting go itself. Awareness releases its
death grip on states, perceptions, and feelings when it sees what
they actually are.

LETTING THE CHAOS ROLL

The experience of illness reveals the chaotic nature of all these
different components of experience, doesn't it? When we have
energy, health, and a reasonable amount of pleasant feeling on
the physical level, we can maintain a degree of personal control
with regard to the *khandas*. Although absolute control is illu-
sory, it is possible to exert our will just enough to feel like we've
got everything neatly packaged within parameters we deem acceptable. Hooked into the energy of becoming, our attention
constellates around various self-views of who we feel we are,
what we want to look like, and how we always will be. This is

the default strategy of the ego. For all of us, the cracks in this illusion are always there. When we are ill for any significant length of time, they become too wide to plaster over. A deeper surrender is required. If we look with wisdom and a real interest in true freedom, we notice that these cracks in the mind's ideals about "my life" are not wrong—they are a fundamental characteristic of human experience. While it is essential to attend to the feelings of disappointment and frustration, loneliness and grief, that arise whenever we are initiated into this surrender, there is another side to it as well. When our personal will is frustrated by limitation and pain or the failure to be the person we wanted to be, we have an opportunity to look deeper into the nature of experience. If we relax the tightness of hankering after "what could have been," we begin to see what actually is: a flow of conditions that are ultimately out of our personal control. We didn't make this body. We didn't make this mind. They are just here, miraculously. What happens when we let go of the illusion of being the head honcho, in charge of it all, personally to blame for it all, and instead let go into a quiet yet curious surrender? Whenever I am inducted (often reluctantly) into this process—through failure and another day of frustrated desire—I remember once again that it is possible to make peace with chaos. It is nature. When attention isn't looking for a center to hold onto in terms of a self-view or a world measuring me according to who I should be, even conventionally unwanted experiences can be felt as part of this mysterious Ferris wheel of change. Where does it arise from? Where does it disappear to? There is of course no answer to these questions; they point to an attitude of wonder and intimacy with conditions that emerge when we let go of trying to force experience into a mold of how it should be. In the process, our real life begins to shine forth from behind conditions. We realize that the death grip on conditions is actually what kills the possibility for harmony, inner vitality, and a truly creative response to life. Surrendering to chaos, free of identification with it, opens a door to this possibility in the core of our being. Paradoxically, you may find it has a healing effect on certain conditions at the same time. Abiding with a heart of letting go will also allow you to intuit deeper truths about both your mind and the way you need to live in order to be as well as you can be—many of which are obscured when the heart is knotted up in a tight ball of anxiety, bitterness, or frantic efforts to package experience into a neat box. While the ego-mind thinks those strategies are leading to well-being, they are actually obstructing it on a deeper level.

Learning this art of surrender takes both time and wisdom. Like all aspects of this inner art, it involves a process of trial and error. You may find yourself letting go too much (without a stable foundation in awareness) and becoming lost in lassitude or passivity, then rebounding into tightness, control, or becoming obsessed with only one outcome. This is a natural kind of swinging—one I have been through countless times. The art of letting go involves surrendering out of any position at all. And yet it is not at odds with positions, agendas, or relative strategies. We can pick them up and then let them go. So it leads to a dynamic responsiveness—we want to get well, but we don't cling tightly to that desire. We don't resist un-wellness. We allow our desire for healing and well-being to come from a place that is in tune with the actual facts of experience rather than a fantasy of "me" expanding into more and more health and pleasant feeling within an eternal paradise on earth. So far, that hasn't worked out for anyone.

THE FACT OF DEATH

In many ways, a life lived with ongoing illness involves a lot of death already. On the micro level, there is always something to die out of. We die out of the life we would have been living "if we weren't ill." We die out of the job we could have done if we had more energy. We die out of the social scene we were once a part of. These tiny deaths are always going on, perhaps under the radar of our everyday awareness. If we look, we see how the *khandas* associated with futures, ideals, and identities also die in the process. For example, when I wake up in discomfort and pain, having finally fallen asleep at five in the morning, it is often the case that the mind that had been holding a perception of myself and "who I would be today" hits up against a wall. In order to make a decision in line with conditions and in harmony with self-care, that perception needs to be let go of. That self-view dies. In the process of writing this book, the "me who can write words about practicing with illness" has died countless times. I have spent weeks completely unable to access the part of the mind that can even begin to form words about this topic. That mind just dies. Right in the middle of that, however, nature is revealing itself—if I listen. As I sit there, staring out of the window, my computer humming away waiting for words to be written, I have two choices. First, I can fight the process and try to resurrect the "writing me" before it is time. This is usually a disaster. The failure to do so leads to frustration, feelings of failure, and an undercurrent of despair. Underlying this kind of relationship to the death of mental states is a mind that has missed the fact of impermanence. It assumes states and capacities should have been permanent. It freaks out when they vanish. The other option has a different quality to it. It comes when I let the moment be exactly as it is. I can notice, "Oh, the writing me has died today. Look at that. It's just . . . gone." In that direct seeing there is also trust that it will return when conditions are right. The deal is that I let go. This trust feels peaceful. It is not based on my personal will—getting things when and how I want them—but rather a much more spacious resting in the awareness that remains mysteriously present, even as states and capacities change, flow, die, and come back to life. Allowing this kind of everyday death allows me to live. Although it sometimes also involves directly being with grief, worry, and fear, the letting go of control at the heart of it is liberating and quietly clears the ground for creativity whenever it wants to return.

If you have lived with illness for any length of time, you are probably intimately familiar with this process. Being consciously alive involves living harmoniously with death already, doesn't it? If we are to be truly aware and responsive to the flow of conditions, particularly the ones that bring challenges and pain, we are called to allow the natural cycles of everyday birth and death to be as they are. This allowing frees the mind and relieves our heart.

For all of us, the physical death of this body will be the ultimate letting go. None of us can avoid it as much as we may subconsciously assume we can. While the stream of our culture generally flows in the direction of wishing never to age, never to experience loss, and to hold on as tightly as possible to what is "mine," it is possible to reflect on the sober facts of mortality in a way that gives us both meaning and perspective on the present moment. At some point everything we know, love, and take to be ourselves will vanish. Living in the light of this recognition allows us to let go more freely. We recognize that nothing is ultimately ours to begin with. Our identity, possessions, and relationships are all temporary. Really taking this into the heart is breathtaking. It inspires a sense of awe and wakes us up to the preciousness of what we do have. When I recollect the transience of all of this—the ones I love, the person I take myself to be—it opens the heart to a deeper perspective than the particular concerns of the storytelling mind. It uncovers a sacredness underneath each moment. Realizing the fragility of all of experience, we start to touch it more gently and hold it with greater love.

So the recollection of our own mortality is useful for all of us, healthy or ill. The Buddha called the contemplation of death the King of Meditations, as it quickens something deep in our being that can let go of all the layers of apparent reality and apparent meaning that attention is so readily consumed by on a day-to-day level. Rather than speculating about what may or may not happen after death, we can use the fact of death to unbind awareness from all that is impermanent and uncover an abiding place of peace in the heart right now. Whatever beliefs your everyday mind has about death, they are just what they are. In the light of this contemplation, however, they can be viewed as aspects of the *khandas:* perceptions, thoughts, and even feelings or intuitions that arise and cease in this moment. It doesn't mean you have to get rid of them or that they don't have their uses. It's about unpacking and unfolding the tenacious, primal habit of selfing that calcifies around the assumption of permanence.

Attending to the inevitability of death in this direct way can take you right back into silent awareness right now. It can include everything. The Buddha himself sometimes described this fundamental principle of awareness as being "deathless" (*amata* in Pali), and "unconstructed" (*asankhata* in Pali). While these words have been subject to countless intellectual disputes over the millennia as to what they "really mean," they are are merely pointers. Unbinding the heart and tasting peace is the point. Words are just there to support that.

I have no idea what happens after the body dies. Whenever I think about the fact that it will one day happen to me, it blows my mind. It is unfathomable. Whatever beliefs I have about it, I can't back them up with evidence-based research. No one who has died is around to talk about it anymore. If we are honest, it remains the ultimate mystery for all of us. When I bring this to mind, I am struck by the mystery of life itself, right here and now. What is *this* anyway? There are so many things we take to be real, important, absolutely true—and yet in the light of death they too are known to be impermanent.

While we can never know for sure what the experience will be when the life force leaves this body of ours, we can contemplate death in a way that liberates the heart and puts our life into perspective. When done at the right time, with an open heart and a genuinely inquisitive mind, it gives awareness the power to come back to that which is reliable and immutable right now: awareness itself. There is great peace in that. We can ask ourselves, in our heart of hearts, "What is it that isn't changing right now? What doesn't leave? What will be a refuge as the body is fading and everything I have known and loved disappears?"

These questions are not aimed toward finding an answer on the conceptual level. Their purpose is to invite us to look, to inquire and peel back the veils of the mind for ourselves. The aim of contemplating death with pure awareness is not to come up with a belief system or to understand, predict, or know anything about what might happen after death through thought. It is to visualize what it will be like for all of us when everything conditioned ceases, and to let that fact take us deeply into awareness itself right now. Let it quicken something deep within you—deeper than ideas, deeper than certainties. Done wisely and with sensitivity, it brings us back home into a profound silence, trust, and peace that cannot be quantified by the thinking mind. It just is.

MEDITATION ON DEATH

If you find uncomfortable energies such as doubt, fear, or grief become overwhelming while doing this practice, then the best thing to do is stop and come back to self-compassion and a feeling of trust that everything is OK. It is all right for some fear to become conscious in the process. Sometimes you will be in the

space to hold it in a way that points you to where you are clinging, while at other times you may need to wisely direct your attention to something else—something that calms and brightens
your heart. The point of this meditation is not to freak you out.
It is to come back home to the peace underneath everything impermanent in this moment.

Take a few moments to connect to the rhythm of breathing—
your trusty, ever-present companion. Feel the breath directly in
your whole body. Make space for it. Enjoy it.

When you feel settled and present, bring the fact of death
into awareness; the fact that this life of ours is finite. What does
that mean? Ask the question in your heart of hearts. Gently put
aside explanations, theories, and ideas. Feel the question. Breathe
with it. Let it touch you.

Consciously let in the reality that everything you have, you
are, you own, you know, will one day cease. Take a few moments to really contemplate this. In this light, what aspects of
your life seem less weighty—more trivial or insignificant perhaps? What kind of perspective does the recollection of this fact
bring to the ups and downs of illness, the failures, disappoint-
ments, and disabilities? Take some time to get a feeling for this
shift of perspective.

Now, with sensitivity and trust in your own resource of
equanimity and self-compassion, imagine that you have only
one week to live. What would that be like? Really imagine that
this is the case. Take as long as you need to let in the immensity
of that and the initial disorientation it may bring about. This is
not bad. It can be used to reorient the heart right now.

Bring the finite nature of all of experience—the body, relationships, feelings, stories, identities, roles, judgments—into full
consciousness. Everything known, identified with, tangible, and
familiar will cease. Without going into more stories, inquire into

the fact of your innate awareness itself. Is it still here when you imagine going through this scenario? What is left when there is no story, no time, no concern, no burden, no ideas, no mask, no illness? Can you sense a purity to awareness when it rests simply as itself? What is it like to surrender into that? What does it take to open the hand of the heart? What happens when it opens?

These are your own questions. Sit with them, revisit them, let them open you up to a whole new perspective on life.

LETTING GO INTO LIFE

Whatever shifts occur for you when you delve deeply into this meditation, it is important not to cling to the aftereffects they produce either. Letting go is a dynamic process and always involves a conscious relationship to *this* moment. This willingness to be in relationship with the moment is the paradox of really tasting impermanence. We know that no idea, perspective, or belief will free the heart. Those are ephemeral too. Holding tightly to an idea of "it's all impermanent" can actually become an obstruction to really availing oneself to the taste in the very moment itself. The point is not to dissociate from our lives but rather to learn a way to relate to our illness wisely. While bringing awareness to the facts of impermanence, the cycles of death within life—and our mortality itself—open up a space in ourselves that sees conditions in their true perspective, it never means denying or pretending that they are not present. So allowing impermanence involves relating to them wisely as they arise, sustain, and cease. Deep insights and moments of clarity all have residues of good feeling, expansiveness, and peace. But those residues cannot be clung to. The real peace is something that sneaks up on us. It begins to permeate all of the myriad states we find ourselves in, difficult or fortunate. It is a result of not only allowing the fact of change, ceasing, and death, but the fact of life as well. Allowing our life to be exactly as it is right now always involves dying out of the ideas we have about how it should be. Letting go is letting life be.

About the Author

PETER FERNANDO lived as a Buddhist monk in the Thai Forest tradition for seven years, his main training being under Ajahn Pasanno and Ajahn Amaro at Abhayagiri Monastery in Redwood Valley, California. Upon leaving the monastic life he was invited to teach by the mindfulness trainer and meditation teacher Stephen Archer and was one of the founders of Original Nature Meditation Centre in Wellington, New Zealand.

Having lived with chronic pain and various health problems himself, Peter has been working with others in similar situations, on an individual basis in Wellington and Auckland, New Zealand, and in groups through the Wellington Multiple Sclerosis Society. He is interested in the intersection between contemporary somatic practices and traditional frameworks for cultivating insight and awakening the heart. One of the main focuses of his practice and teaching in this area is a reframing of views around illness from those of shame and self-criticism to compassion and open-hearted exploration.

Peter is enthusiastic about the possibility of fostering a sense of community and support online for those who cannot attend groups in person. In addition to his work in person in New Zealand, he has been teaching internationally since 2011 through an online meditation course called "A Month of Mindfulness": www.monthofmindfulness.info.